Mental Health and Well Being

Jagdish Krishanlal Arora

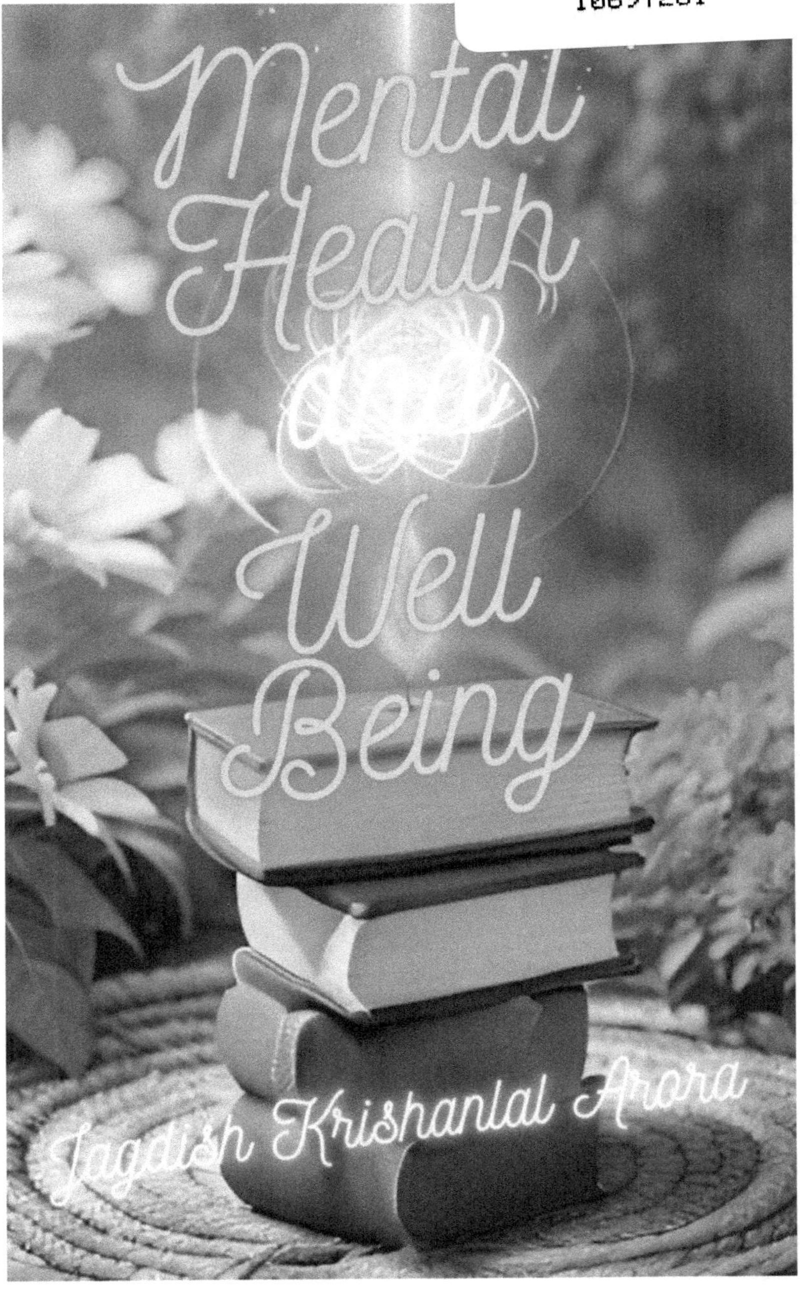

MENTAL HEALTH AND WELL BEING
BY
JAGDISH KRISHANLAL ARORA

This is a work of fiction. Similarities to real people, places, or events are entirely coincidental.

MENTAL HEALTH AND WELL BEING

First edition. October 2, 2023.

Copyright © 2023 Jagdish Krishanlal Arora.

Written by Jagdish Krishanlal Arora.

Table of Contents

Introduction

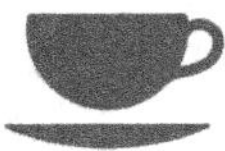

Mental health is a fundamental aspect of human well-being that influences every facet of our lives. It shapes our thoughts, emotions, behaviors, relationships, and overall quality of life. Yet, despite its paramount importance, mental health often remains in the shadows, misunderstood, stigmatized, and even ignored. This chapter endeavors to shed light on the intricate tapestry of mental health, unraveling its essence, significance, the multifaceted factors that mold it, the prevalent disorders that challenge it, the stigma that shrouds it, and the constructive strategies to nurture and preserve it.

In a world where the pursuit of physical health is ceaseless, mental health frequently languishes in the periphery. It's time to rectify this oversight, for just as our bodies require care and attention, so too do our minds. In exploring the depths of mental health, we embark on a journey to unveil its profound impact on our lives. It is the cornerstone upon which our thoughts take shape, our emotions find resonance, our behaviors emerge, and our relationships flourish or falter. It is the invisible hand that guides the ship of our existence, often steering us through calm waters, but occasionally navigating us through treacherous storms.

Yet, mental health remains enigmatic to many. What exactly is it? Why is it so critical? What factors conspire to mold it? What happens when it falters, giving rise to the often-daunting realm of mental disorders? How can we combat the stigma that shrouds discussions of mental health? What practical steps can we take to promote and safeguard our mental well-being? These are the questions that beckon answers, and it is the purpose of this chapter to provide them.

In the pages that follow, we will venture into the heart of mental health, not as a distant and abstract concept, but as an integral part of our daily lives. We will seek to demystify it, breaking down the barriers of misconception and prejudice. We will acknowledge that mental health is not an outlier or an anomaly; it is the very essence of our humanity. Understanding it is not a luxury but a necessity. It is the compass that guides us towards a fulfilling and harmonious existence, helping us to navigate life's challenges and savor its joys.

Chapter 1- What is Mental Health?

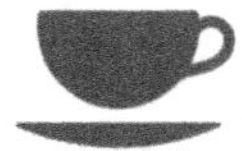

Mental health, often relegated to the shadows of our consciousness, is an intricate tapestry of our emotional, psychological, and social well-being. It constitutes the very essence of our humanity, influencing the trajectory of our lives in ways both subtle and profound. At its core, mental health is about more than just the absence of mental disorders; it is a state of profound equilibrium where an individual's inner world harmonizes with their outer experiences.

Picture it as the conductor of an orchestra, orchestrating the symphony of our thoughts, emotions, behaviors, and relationships. It determines whether this symphony is a harmonious melody or a discordant cacophony. When mental health is robust, it equips us with the tools to navigate life's tempestuous waters with resilience and grace. It is the sturdy vessel that allows us to weather storms, adapt to change, and emerge from adversity not broken but strengthened.

In its most tangible form, good mental health is the ability to manage stress, to hold the delicate threads of relationships without letting them unravel, to engage in productive work, and to make decisions rooted in reason rather than impulsivity. It is the capacity to find joy in the mundane, to appreciate the beauty of existence, and to savor the moments of connection with others.

But mental health is not a static state; it's dynamic, ever-evolving, and exquisitely sensitive to the currents of life. It's the pendulum that swings between moments of triumph and tribulation, between calm and chaos. Just as our bodies fluctuate in health, so too do our minds. And just as we diligently care for our physical well-being, so should we tend to our mental health.

In understanding mental health, we must appreciate that it's not an isolated concept. It's interwoven with every facet of our existence. It's the silent partner in our daily routines, our ambitions, our dreams, and our fears. It's the hidden force that shapes our responses to life's challenges, molds our perspectives, and influences our interactions with others.

So, let us recognize that mental health is not a luxury but a fundamental human right. It is the keystone that supports our pursuit of happiness, fulfillment, and self-actualization. It is the blueprint for a life lived not merely in survival but in thriving. As we delve deeper into the realm of mental health, we will unravel its significance, explore the factors that shape it, confront the disorders that challenge it, and ultimately emerge with a richer understanding of this vital aspect of our lives.

Chapter 2 - The Importance of Mental Health

Mental health is not an abstract concept; it is a cornerstone of our overall well-being. It exerts a profound influence on every aspect of our lives, from our individual well-being to our interpersonal relationships, productivity, and even our physical health. Recognizing the pivotal role that mental health plays in our existence is the first step toward embracing its importance.

A. Individual Well-being

Imagine mental health as the invisible guardian of your well-being, standing by your side as you navigate the labyrinth of life. When it is robust and nurtured, it empowers you to experience life's highs and lows with grace and resilience. Here's why individual well-being hinges on good mental health:

Resilience: Good mental health equips you with the tools to bounce back from adversity. It's the inner strength that helps you weather storms, adapt to change, and emerge from challenges stronger than before.

Effective Stress Management: Life is filled with stressors, both big and small. Good mental health enables you to manage stress effectively, preventing it from overwhelming you or causing chronic health issues.

Emotional Regulation: It provides the ability to navigate a wide spectrum of emotions, from joy to sorrow, anger to serenity, in a healthy and balanced manner. You can appreciate the beauty of joy and cope with the challenges of sorrow without being overwhelmed.

Positive Outlook: With good mental health, you're more likely to maintain a positive outlook on life. You can find joy in the everyday and cultivate an attitude of gratitude.

B. Interpersonal Relationships

Our lives are interwoven with a complex tapestry of relationships. Mental health is the invisible thread that binds these relationships together and influences our ability to connect with others:

Effective Communication: Good mental health enhances your ability to communicate effectively. It allows you to express yourself clearly, listen empathetically, and understand the emotions of those around you.

Empathy: Empathy, the capacity to understand and share the feelings of others, flourishes in a mind that is well. It fosters deep connections and helps build meaningful relationships.

Conflict Resolution: When conflicts inevitably arise, good mental health provides you with the emotional intelligence and problem-solving skills needed to navigate them constructively.

C. Productivity

Mental health is not confined to the boundaries of our personal lives; it extends its reach into our productivity, both in our personal pursuits and in the professional realm:

Focus and Creativity: A person with good mental health is more likely to be focused, creative, and innovative. A well-balanced mind is a fertile ground for generating new ideas and achieving goals.

Efficiency: Productivity and efficiency go hand in hand with mental health. When you're mentally well, you can tackle tasks with clarity and efficiency, achieving more in less time.

D. Physical Health

The connection between mental and physical health is undeniable. Mental health issues can manifest as physical symptoms and contribute to a range of health conditions:

Stress-Related Illnesses: Prolonged mental stress can lead to physical health issues such as heart disease, high blood pressure, and digestive disorders.

Immune Function: Mental health can influence the immune system's effectiveness, impacting the body's ability to defend against infections and illnesses.

Lifestyle Choices: Our mental well-being often guides our lifestyle choices, including diet, exercise, and substance use, all of which have profound implications for our physical health.

In essence, mental health is the invisible thread that weaves through the fabric of our lives, influencing our individual well-being, our ability to connect with others, our productivity, and even the state of our physical health. It is not a luxury but a fundamental aspect of our existence that deserves attention, care, and nurturing. Recognizing its significance is the first step toward embracing a life that is not merely lived but truly thrives.

Chapter 3 - Factors Influencing Mental Health

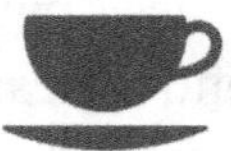

Mental health is a complex tapestry woven from various threads, each representing a different factor that influences its delicate balance. Understanding these factors is crucial for comprehending the intricacies of mental well-being. Here are the key factors that shape our mental health:

A. Biological Factors

At the very core of our mental health lie biological factors, intricately intertwined with our genetic makeup and brain chemistry. These elements can significantly affect how we experience and manage mental health:

Genetics: The genetic lottery plays a role in mental health. Some individuals may inherit a predisposition to mental health disorders, making them more vulnerable to certain conditions. However, genetics alone do not determine mental health outcomes; they interact with other factors.

Brain Chemistry: Neurotransmitters and brain chemicals influence our moods and emotions. Imbalances in these chemicals can contribute to mental health disorders, such as depression and anxiety.

B. Environmental Factors

The environments we inhabit, particularly during critical developmental periods, can leave lasting imprints on our mental health:

Childhood Experiences: Childhood trauma, abuse, neglect, or adverse experiences can have profound and enduring effects on mental health. These early-life experiences can shape our emotional well-being and coping mechanisms in adulthood.

Exposure to Violence: Living in environments where violence is prevalent can cause chronic stress and anxiety, impacting mental health. Witnessing or experiencing violence can lead to conditions like post-traumatic stress disorder (PTSD).

C. Lifestyle and Behavior

Our daily choices and behaviors play a pivotal role in maintaining mental health. These include:

Diet: A balanced diet rich in essential nutrients supports brain health and emotional well-being. Nutritional deficiencies can contribute to mood disorders.

Physical Activity: Regular exercise not only benefits physical health but also has a profound impact on mental health. It can reduce symptoms of depression and anxiety and improve overall well-being.

Substance Use: Substance abuse, including alcohol and drugs, can severely impair mental health. It can exacerbate existing mental health conditions and lead to addiction.

D. Social Support

Our connections with others, our social networks, and the quality of our relationships are critical factors in mental health:

Friends and Family: Strong, supportive relationships with friends and family provide emotional resilience. Having a network of trusted individuals to lean on during difficult times can mitigate the impact of stress and adversity.

Social Isolation: Conversely, social isolation and loneliness are detrimental to mental health. Lack of social connections can lead to feelings of depression and anxiety.

E. Socioeconomic Factors

Socioeconomic status, education, and access to resources also wield substantial influence over mental health:

Economic Hardship: Financial stressors and economic hardship can increase the risk of mental health disorders. The struggle to make ends meet can lead to chronic stress and anxiety.

Access to Mental Health Care: Disparities in access to mental health care and resources can profoundly affect mental health outcomes. Limited access to quality care can delay diagnosis and treatment.

In essence, mental health is the result of a delicate interplay between genetics, biology, life experiences, lifestyle choices, social connections, and socioeconomic circumstances. These factors do not operate in isolation but are interconnected, shaping our mental well-being in complex ways. Recognizing the role each factor plays can guide efforts to promote mental health and provide support to those in need.

Chapter 4 - Common Mental Health Disorders

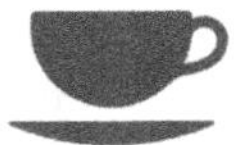

Mental health disorders are a diverse spectrum of conditions that can affect individuals of all ages, backgrounds, and walks of life. These disorders often disrupt an individual's thoughts, emotions, behaviors, and daily functioning. Understanding them is essential for promoting awareness, compassion, and effective treatment. Here are some common mental health disorders:

A. Depression

Characteristics: Depression is marked by persistent feelings of sadness, hopelessness, and a loss of interest or pleasure in activities once enjoyed. Individuals with depression may experience changes in appetite, sleep patterns, and energy levels. Feelings of worthlessness and thoughts of self-harm or suicide can also be present.

Impact: Depression can be debilitating, affecting every aspect of an individual's life. It can disrupt relationships, hinder work or school performance, and lead to physical symptoms like fatigue and aches.

B. Anxiety Disorders

Characteristics: Anxiety disorders encompass a range of conditions, including generalized anxiety disorder, panic disorder, and social anxiety disorder. These disorders are characterized by excessive and irrational worry or fear. Physical symptoms such as rapid heartbeat, sweating, and trembling are common during anxiety episodes.

Impact: Anxiety disorders can interfere with daily life, causing significant distress and impairing an individual's ability to function normally. They may lead to avoidance of certain situations or activities.

C. Bipolar Disorder

Characteristics: Bipolar disorder involves extreme mood swings, cycling between episodes of mania and depression. During manic episodes, individuals may experience elevated mood, increased energy, impulsivity, and decreased need for sleep. Depressive episodes mirror the characteristics of clinical depression.

Impact: Bipolar disorder can disrupt personal relationships, work, and daily routines. Managing mood swings and maintaining stability can be challenging.

D. Schizophrenia

Characteristics: Schizophrenia is a severe mental disorder marked by distorted thinking, hallucinations, delusions, and impaired perception of reality. Individuals with schizophrenia may experience disorganized speech and behavior.

Impact: Schizophrenia can have a profound impact on an individual's life, making it difficult to maintain relationships, employment, and independent living. Treatment and support are essential for managing symptoms.

E. Eating Disorders

Characteristics: Eating disorders include conditions like anorexia nervosa, characterized by extreme restriction of food intake leading to dangerously low body weight, and bulimia nervosa, involving binge eating followed by purging behaviors such as vomiting or excessive exercise.

Impact: Eating disorders can have serious physical and psychological consequences, including malnutrition, heart problems, and damage to vital organs. These disorders often lead to social isolation and a poor quality of life.

These common mental health disorders represent just a fraction of the diverse array of conditions that individuals may experience. It's important to note that mental health disorders are treatable, and individuals living with them can lead fulfilling lives with the right support, treatment, and understanding from their communities. By increasing awareness and reducing stigma surrounding mental health, we can better support those in need and promote overall well-being.

Chapter 5 - Stigma and Mental Health

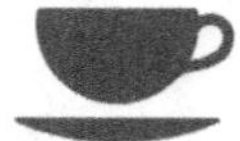

In the intricate landscape of mental health, a formidable barrier often stands between individuals and the help they need: stigma. Mental health stigma is a pervasive, corrosive force that has far-reaching consequences. It weaves a web of discrimination, misunderstanding, and fear that shrouds discussions of mental health in silence and shame.

Stigma: A Formidable Foe

At its core, stigma is a collection of negative beliefs, attitudes, and stereotypes surrounding mental health issues. It's the insidious notion that mental disorders are somehow different from physical ailments, that they are less valid, less real, or even a sign of personal weakness. It's the whispered judgment that those who seek help for their mental health are somehow flawed, broken, or incapable of handling their own lives.

The Consequences of Stigma

The impact of stigma on individuals and society as a whole is profound. Stigma breeds silence, leading many to suffer in silence rather than seek the support they desperately need. It can prevent individuals from disclosing their struggles to friends, family, or coworkers, perpetuating a cycle of isolation and loneliness.

In the broader context, stigma can also influence public policy and resource allocation, often resulting in inadequate support for mental health services. This lack of funding and attention can leave millions without access to the care and resources necessary for recovery.

Combatting Stigma

Understanding and addressing stigma is paramount for promoting mental health awareness and reducing the negative impact of stereotypes. It requires a multifaceted approach:

1. Education: The foundation for dismantling stigma is education. Society must be informed about mental health, its prevalence, and the fact that it can affect anyone, regardless of age, gender, or background. By dispelling myths and fostering understanding, we can begin to break down the walls of stigma.

2. Open Dialogue: Encouraging open and honest conversations about mental health is crucial. When individuals feel safe discussing their struggles, they are more likely to seek help and support. By sharing our experiences and vulnerabilities, we demonstrate that mental health is an intrinsic part of the human experience.

3. Challenging Stereotypes: Stigmatizing stereotypes are deeply ingrained in society. Challenging and confronting these stereotypes when we encounter them is essential. This may involve speaking up when we hear stigmatizing language or correcting misconceptions about mental health.

4. Advocacy: Advocacy at both the individual and societal levels is vital. Individuals can advocate for themselves by seeking help and sharing their stories. On a larger scale, mental health advocates work to influence policy, reduce stigma in the workplace, and improve access to mental health services.

5. Compassion and Empathy: Perhaps most importantly, we must approach mental health with compassion and empathy. Mental health challenges can affect anyone, and no one should ever be made to feel ashamed or isolated because of their struggles. By extending understanding and support, we can create a more inclusive and compassionate society.

Mental health stigma is a formidable adversary, but it is not invincible. With education, open dialogue, challenging stereotypes, advocacy, and above all, compassion and empathy, we can chip away at the foundations of stigma. By doing so, we create a world where seeking help for mental health is not a sign of weakness but an act of courage and self-care. Reducing stigma is not just a goal; it is a necessity for the well-being of individuals and society as a whole.

7. Promoting Mental Well-being

Promoting mental well-being is a proactive and essential approach to maintaining good mental health. Just as we invest time and effort in our physical well-being, nurturing our mental health through deliberate strategies is equally vital. Here are key strategies to foster mental well-being:

A. Self-care

Self-care is the foundation upon which mental well-being is built. It involves a range of practices and behaviors that prioritize your mental and emotional health:

Regular Exercise: Physical activity not only benefits the body but also has a profound impact on mental health. It releases endorphins, reduces stress, and improves mood.

Balanced Diet: Nutrition plays a significant role in mental health. A well-balanced diet with essential nutrients supports brain health and emotional well-being.

Adequate Sleep: Quality sleep is crucial for mental well-being. Poor sleep can lead to mood disturbances and decreased cognitive function.

Mindfulness and Meditation: Mindfulness practices, such as meditation and deep breathing exercises, can help you stay grounded, reduce stress, and enhance emotional resilience.

John's journey towards mental well-being is a testament to the enduring nature of this pursuit. As a retired teacher, he had spent a significant portion of his life helping students navigate the challenges of academia and life. However, it was only in retirement that he truly began to appreciate the importance of his own mental health.

The Early Retirement Years

John's journey began with retirement, a time many look forward to as a period of relaxation and enjoyment. However, John found himself facing a sense of emptiness and restlessness. The structured routine of teaching was suddenly gone, leaving a void he hadn't anticipated.

Recognizing the Need for Change

After a few months of aimlessness, John recognized that something needed to change. He realized that, just like his students had needed guidance and support, he needed to provide the same for himself. Mental health, he understood, wasn't something to be taken for granted.

Exploring New Avenues

John began his journey to mental well-being by exploring new interests and hobbies. He joined a local art class, started reading books he'd always wanted to read but never had the time for, and even began volunteering at a nearby community center. These activities not only filled his time but also provided him with a sense of purpose and connection to others.

The Role of Mindfulness

As he goes deeper into his journey, John discovered the power of mindfulness. He started attending mindfulness meditation sessions and practicing mindfulness on his own. Mindfulness allowed him to be fully present in each moment, to appreciate the beauty of life around him, and to let go of unnecessary worries about the past and future.

Building Social Connections

Recognizing the importance of social connections, John rekindled old friendships and made new ones. He realized that nurturing relationships was a vital part of mental well-being. Regular meet-ups with friends and participating in group activities not only brought joy into his life but also provided a support system during challenging times.

Facing Setbacks

John's journey wasn't without setbacks. There were days when he felt overwhelmed by the uncertainties of life, the passing of time, and the challenges of aging. During these moments, he turned to the resilience-building strategies he had learned. He reminded himself of the progress he had made and the resilience he had developed over time.

The Ongoing Odyssey

As John reflects on his journey, he emphasizes that mental health is a lifelong pursuit. It's not a destination one arrives at but a continuous effort to nurture and care for one's well-being. Each step taken, whether big or small, brings him closer to a happier and healthier life.

John's story is a reminder that mental well-being is not something that can be achieved and forgotten; it's an ongoing process. It requires self-awareness, self-compassion, and a commitment to personal growth. John's journey inspires us to embark on our own path towards mental well-being, knowing that every step we take is a step towards a more fulfilling and resilient life.

B. Building Resilience

Resilience is the ability to adapt and bounce back from adversity. It's a valuable skill that can be cultivated over time:

Problem-Solving Skills: Developing effective problem-solving skills can help you navigate challenges more successfully. It involves breaking down problems into manageable steps and seeking solutions.

Emotional Regulation: Understanding and managing your emotions is essential for resilience. Practices like journaling or talking to a therapist can help you process difficult emotions.

Positive Thinking: Cultivating a positive outlook can boost resilience. Focus on your strengths and achievements, and practice gratitude.

Emma's journey is a powerful testament to the strength of the human spirit and the remarkable capacity for resilience in the face of adversity. Her story serves as an inspiring example of how resilience can help individuals overcome even the darkest of times.

The Traumatic Accident

Emma's life took a drastic turn on a fateful day when she was involved in a traumatic accident. The physical and emotional scars from the incident were profound, and the journey towards recovery appeared daunting and insurmountable.

The Initial Struggles

In the immediate aftermath of the accident, Emma grappled with intense physical pain and emotional trauma. The physical rehabilitation process was demanding, requiring immense patience and determination. Yet, it was the emotional scars that proved to be the most challenging aspect of her recovery.

The Power of Resilience

Emma's journey towards healing was marked by her unwavering resilience. She refused to succumb to despair and self-pity. Instead, she embarked on a path of self-discovery and healing. She sought the guidance of mental health professionals who helped her navigate the complex terrain of trauma and its aftermath.

Seeking Support

A crucial aspect of Emma's journey was seeking and accepting support from her loved ones. She learned the importance of vulnerability and how sharing her experiences and feelings with others could alleviate the burden she carried. Her friends and family became pillars of strength, offering unwavering support and love.

Therapeutic Techniques

Emma also explored various therapeutic techniques to aid her healing process. Mindfulness meditation, in particular, played a significant role in helping her manage the intrusive thoughts and flashbacks that often haunted her. By learning to stay present in the moment, she gradually gained more control over her emotions.

The Role of Acceptance

Acceptance was another pivotal aspect of Emma's journey. She came to terms with the fact that her life had changed irreversibly due to the accident. Rather than dwelling on what was lost, she focused on what she could still achieve and experience. This shift in perspective was transformative.

Small Steps Toward Recovery

Emma's recovery was not linear. There were setbacks and difficult days. However, she understood that healing wasn't about reaching a fixed destination but about the journey itself. She celebrated the small victories, no matter how insignificant they may have seemed to others.

Becoming a Source of Inspiration

Over time, Emma's resilience and determination began to inspire those around her. Her story served as a beacon of hope for others who faced adversity. She became involved in support groups and advocacy work, sharing her experiences and offering guidance to others on their own journeys to recovery.

The Ongoing Journey

Emma's journey continues, a testament to the enduring nature of resilience. She acknowledges that healing is not a one-time event but a lifelong process. By embracing the challenges and uncertainties of life, she has discovered a profound sense of strength and purpose.

Emma's story reminds us that resilience is not the absence of pain or adversity but the ability to bounce back and grow stronger in the face of it. Her journey is a shining example of how, with resilience, support, and self-compassion, one can overcome even the darkest of times and emerge from them as a beacon of inspiration for others. Emma's story underscores the indomitable spirit of the human heart and the capacity for healing and growth that resides within each of us.

C. Seeking Social Support

Maintaining meaningful relationships and seeking support from friends and family during times of distress is a cornerstone of mental well-being:

Healthy Relationships: Nurture and invest in your relationships. Engage in open communication, active listening, and empathetic understanding. Healthy relationships provide a source of emotional support.

Seeking Help: Don't hesitate to seek professional help when needed. Mental health professionals can provide guidance, therapy, and tools for managing mental health challenges.

D. Reducing Stress

Stress is a natural part of life, but effective stress management is essential for mental well-being:

Time Management: Organize your time and prioritize tasks to reduce feelings of overwhelm. Time management techniques can help you achieve a sense of control over your daily life.

Relaxation Exercises: Incorporate relaxation techniques into your routine, such as deep breathing exercises, progressive muscle relaxation, or yoga. These practices can reduce stress and promote relaxation.

Set Boundaries: Establish clear boundaries in your personal and professional life to prevent burnout and maintain a healthy work-life balance.

Promoting mental well-being is an ongoing journey that requires attention and effort. By integrating these strategies into your daily life, you can create a strong foundation for mental health and resilience. Remember that mental well-being is not a destination but a continuous process of self-care and growth.

8. Seeking Help and Treatment

One of the most crucial steps in the journey towards better mental health is recognizing when you need help and taking action to seek it. Mental health challenges are not a sign of weakness or failure, but a part of the human experience. Fortunately, there are various treatment options and support systems available to assist individuals in managing their mental health effectively.

1. Therapy

Therapy, often referred to as counseling or psychotherapy, is a fundamental and widely recognized form of mental health treatment. It involves talking to a trained mental health professional, such as a psychologist, psychiatrist, social worker, or counselor, in a safe and confidential environment.

Individual Therapy: One-on-one sessions with a therapist allow for personalized discussions and tailored interventions. Cognitive-behavioral therapy (CBT), dialectical-behavior therapy (DBT), and talk therapy are some common approaches.

Group Therapy: Group therapy involves sessions with a small group of individuals facing similar challenges. It can provide a sense of community and shared support.

Family Therapy: In cases where family dynamics significantly impact an individual's mental health, family therapy can be beneficial. It focuses on improving communication and resolving conflicts within the family unit.

2. Medication

In some cases, mental health challenges may benefit from medication prescribed by a psychiatrist or medical doctor. Medications are often used in conjunction with therapy and can help manage symptoms of various conditions, including depression, anxiety disorders, bipolar disorder, and schizophrenia.

It's essential to work closely with a healthcare provider to determine the right medication and dosage, as individual responses can vary. Medication should be taken as prescribed, and any concerns or side effects should be promptly discussed with the prescribing physician.

3. Support Groups

Support groups offer a valuable sense of community and understanding for individuals facing similar mental health challenges. These groups can be facilitated by mental health professionals or peer-led, and they provide a platform for sharing experiences, strategies, and coping mechanisms.

Support groups exist for a wide range of mental health conditions, including addiction recovery, grief and loss, post-traumatic stress disorder (PTSD), and more. Finding a support group that aligns with your needs and preferences can be a significant step toward emotional healing.

4. Online and Telehealth Services

The advent of technology has made mental health services more accessible than ever before. Online therapy platforms and telehealth services allow individuals to connect with mental health professionals remotely. This can be especially beneficial for those with limited access to in-person services or those who prefer the convenience and privacy of virtual sessions.

5. Overcoming Stigma

Seeking help for mental health challenges can be hindered by the stigma that still surrounds mental health issues. It's crucial to remember that seeking help is a sign of strength, not weakness. It takes courage to acknowledge your struggles and reach out for support.

By openly discussing mental health, challenging stereotypes, and sharing personal stories, we can collectively work to reduce the stigma surrounding mental health care. It's a collective responsibility to foster an environment where seeking help for mental health is not only accepted but encouraged.

In conclusion, seeking help and treatment is a vital step on the path to better mental health. It's a declaration that your well-being matters and that you are taking proactive steps to improve your life. Remember that there is no one-size-fits-all approach to mental health treatment; what works best for you may vary. The key is to reach out, explore your options, and find the support and treatment that resonate with your unique needs and circumstances.

Chapter 6 - Analysis of Mental Health

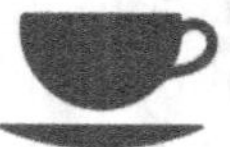

In the complex tapestry of human existence, mental health stands as a vital and often underappreciated thread. Understanding what mental health is, why it matters, and how to nurture it is essential for crafting a life that is not merely lived but truly thrives.

Mental Health: The Bedrock of Well-being

Mental health is not an abstract concept; it's the heartbeat of our well-being. It guides our thoughts, emotions, behaviors, and relationships. It empowers us to face life's challenges with resilience, adaptability, and hope. It's the key to experiencing joy and sorrow, love and loss, and all the intricate emotions that make us human.

The Significance of Mental Health

The significance of mental health is woven into every facet of our lives:

Individual Well-being: It allows us to navigate the highs and lows of life with grace. It equips us to manage stress, maintain a positive outlook, and bounce back from adversity.

Interpersonal Relationships: It's the invisible thread that binds us to others, enabling us to connect, communicate, and empathize.

Productivity: It fuels our creativity, focus, and efficiency in both personal and professional pursuits.

Physical Health: The mind-body connection is undeniable, with mental health influencing physical health outcomes.

Factors at Play

The delicate balance of mental health is influenced by a multitude of factors, from our genetics and biology to our life experiences, lifestyle choices, and social connections. Recognizing the interplay of these factors is essential for understanding the intricacies of mental well-being.

Facing the Shadows: Common Disorders and Stigma

Common mental health disorders, such as depression, anxiety, bipolar disorder, schizophrenia, and eating disorders, are part of the human experience. They do not define us but challenge us to seek help and support when needed.

Yet, stigma often casts a long shadow over these challenges. It perpetuates silence, isolation, and discrimination. Addressing stigma is not just an option; it's a necessity for fostering mental health awareness and building a compassionate society.

Promoting a Brighter Future

Promoting mental well-being is not an idle endeavor but a proactive journey. It involves practicing self-care, building resilience, seeking social support, and managing stress effectively. By embracing these strategies, we can fortify our mental health and lead more fulfilling lives.

A Call to Action

This chapter is not merely a collection of words but a call to action. It's an invitation to recognize the importance of mental health in our lives, to challenge stereotypes, and to support those who need it. Together, we can create a world where mental health is not overshadowed by stigma but celebrated as an integral part of our shared humanity.

In the end, understanding mental health is not a destination but a lifelong journey, a commitment to ourselves and our communities. It's a testament to our resilience, our capacity for growth, and our shared responsibility to create a world where mental health thrives, and every individual has the opportunity to lead a life of purpose, resilience, and well-being.

Chapter 7 - The Importance of Mental Health Exercises

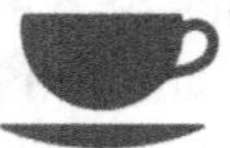

The importance of mental health exercises cannot be overstated in today's fast-paced and often stressful world. In the introductory chapter of a book or program focused on mental health, several key points are typically addressed to establish the significance of these exercises:

Emotional Well-being: The introductory chapter begins by emphasizing the paramount importance of emotional well-being. It explains that mental health is not merely the absence of mental illness but the presence of positive qualities such as resilience, emotional intelligence, and overall psychological well-being.

Prevalence of Mental Health Challenges: It acknowledges the widespread prevalence of mental health challenges, including stress, anxiety, depression, and more. These challenges affect individuals from all walks of life, making it essential to prioritize mental health.

Impact on Physical Health: The chapter may also touch upon the close connection between mental and physical health. It's well-documented that poor mental health can lead to physical health problems and vice versa. This underscores the need for mental health exercises as a proactive approach to overall well-being.

The Role of Exercises: The core message of the chapter is to convey that mental health exercises are powerful tools to address and improve emotional well-being. These exercises can range from mindfulness and meditation practices to cognitive-behavioral techniques and self-care routines.

Scientific Basis: The introductory chapter might briefly mention the scientific basis behind mental health exercises. Research and studies have consistently shown that engaging in these exercises can lead to positive changes in brain function and structure, improved mood, reduced stress, and enhanced resilience.

Practicality: It also emphasizes that the book or program will provide practical, actionable exercises that individuals can incorporate into their daily lives. This makes it clear that improving mental health is not an abstract concept but something achievable through regular practice.

A Holistic Approach: The chapter may highlight the holistic nature of mental health exercises. They not only address immediate concerns but also foster personal growth, improved relationships, and an overall sense of fulfillment.

Personal Responsibility: Lastly, the introductory chapter often encourages readers to take personal responsibility for their mental health. It emphasizes that while external support is valuable, individuals have the power to initiate positive change in their lives through these exercises.

Chapter 8 - The Science Behind Mental Health Exercises

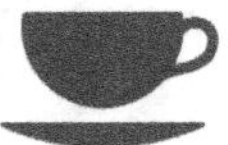

This chapter takes a closer look at the scientific foundations of mental health exercises. We explore the neurological and psychological mechanisms that underlie the effectiveness of these exercises. Through studies and expert insights, we highlight how engaging in mental health exercises can reshape our brain, improve emotional regulation, and boost overall well-being.

In today's fast-paced and demanding world, the pursuit of well-being has become a paramount concern. While physical health often takes the spotlight, mental health is equally vital for leading a fulfilling life. Just as we engage in physical exercises to enhance our physical health, mental health exercises are crucial tools for nurturing and fortifying our psychological well-being. In this chapter, we will embark on a journey to explore the concept of mental health exercises and their profound significance in promoting overall well-being.

Mental health exercises encompass a wide array of practices and techniques designed to enhance mental and emotional fitness. These exercises are not just tools for individuals already struggling with mental health issues; they are proactive steps that anyone can take to boost their mental resilience and maintain a balanced and healthy mind.

Neurological Foundations

Our journey into the realm of mental health exercises begins with understanding the intricate relationship between these practices and our brain. The brain is an astonishingly adaptable organ, capable of reshaping itself in response to new experiences and challenges. This phenomenon is known as neuroplasticity, and it forms the basis of how mental health exercises can effect profound changes in our brain's structure and function.

Neuroplasticity allows the brain to rewire its neural pathways in response to learning and experiences. When we engage in mental health exercises, we stimulate this neuroplasticity, enabling our brain to adapt and change. Specific brain regions and neural pathways are impacted by these exercises, leading to improved cognitive function, emotional regulation, and overall mental well-being.

Psychological Mechanisms

To go deeper into the world of mental health exercises, it is crucial to explore the psychological mechanisms at play. These exercises encompass a variety of practices, including mindfulness, cognitive-behavioral techniques, and positive psychology interventions. They are designed to influence thought patterns, emotions, and behaviors positively.

Mindfulness, for example, encourages us to be present in the moment, fostering self-awareness and reducing the grip of intrusive or negative thoughts. Cognitive-behavioral techniques empower individuals to identify and challenge unhelpful thought patterns, replacing them with healthier alternatives. Positive psychology interventions promote gratitude, optimism, and resilience, ultimately enhancing emotional well-being.

Emotional Regulation

One of the most significant benefits of mental health exercises lies in their capacity to enhance emotional regulation. Emotional regulation refers to our ability to manage and respond to emotions effectively. Mental health exercises equip individuals with the tools to navigate stress, anxiety, and other emotional challenges.

These exercises encourage self-reflection and emotional awareness, enabling individuals to recognize and address the root causes of their emotional struggles. By practicing mindfulness or cognitive-behavioral techniques, individuals can develop healthier coping strategies, reduce emotional reactivity, and foster a greater sense of emotional balance.

Scientific Studies and Evidence

The effectiveness of mental health exercises is not a mere conjecture; it is firmly grounded in scientific research. Numerous studies have provided compelling evidence for the positive impact of these exercises on mental health. Researchers have employed various methodologies to investigate the effects of mindfulness, cognitive-behavioral therapy, and positive psychology interventions on psychological well-being.

For instance, studies have shown that regular mindfulness practice can lead to significant reductions in symptoms of anxiety and depression. Cognitive-behavioral therapy has been demonstrated to be highly effective in treating a range of mental health disorders, from phobias to post-traumatic stress disorder. Positive psychology interventions have been associated with increased levels of happiness and life satisfaction.

Expert Insights

To gain a deeper understanding of the significance of mental health exercises, we turn to the insights of mental health professionals and researchers in the field. These experts provide valuable perspectives on why these exercises are beneficial and shed light on the underlying scientific mechanisms at play.

Dr. Sarah Thompson, a renowned psychologist, emphasizes that mental health exercises empower individuals by enhancing their self-awareness and emotional regulation. She explains that these exercises work by rewiring neural pathways in the brain, promoting healthier thought patterns and behaviors. According to Dr. Thompson, "Engaging in mental health exercises is like giving your brain a workout, and just as physical exercise strengthens your muscles, these exercises strengthen your mental resilience."

Brain Reshaping and Plasticity

The concept of brain reshaping through mental health exercises is a captivating one. It underscores the idea that our brains are not static entities but rather dynamic and adaptable. As we engage in mindfulness, meditation, or other mental health practices, our brains respond by creating new neural connections and reinforcing existing ones.

This process leads to positive changes in the brain's structure and function. For instance, studies have shown that regular meditation can increase gray matter density in brain regions associated with memory, empathy, and stress regulation. Cognitive-behavioral therapy can alter the patterns of activity in the brain regions responsible for processing emotions and decision-making. These changes translate into improved mental well-being and emotional resilience.

Overall Well-being

In summary, our exploration of mental health exercises reveals their profound impact on overall well-being. These exercises, grounded in scientific principles, offer individuals a path to enhanced mental resilience, emotional regulation, and psychological well-being. By stimulating neuroplasticity, rewiring neural pathways, and fostering healthier thought patterns and behaviors, mental health exercises hold the promise of a more balanced and fulfilling life.

Practical Application

To make the knowledge gained in this chapter actionable, here are some practical exercises that readers can incorporate into their daily lives:

Mindful Breathing: Set aside a few minutes each day to engage in mindful breathing. Focus your attention on your breath, inhaling and exhaling slowly. This practice can help reduce stress and increase self-awareness.

Thought Journaling: Keep a journal to record your thoughts and emotions. Identify any negative thought patterns and challenge them with more rational and positive alternatives.

Gratitude Practice: Make a daily habit of listing three things you are grateful for. This simple exercise can boost your mood and enhance your overall outlook on life.

Progressive Muscle Relaxation: Learn and practice progressive muscle relaxation techniques to alleviate physical tension and promote relaxation.

We've embarked on a journey to uncover the transformative power of mental health exercises. We began by introducing the concept and emphasizing their importance in promoting well-being. We explored the neurological foundations, delving into the fascinating realm of neuroplasticity and how mental health exercises impact specific brain regions and neural pathways. Moving on to the psychological mechanisms, we examined how these exercises influence thought patterns and emotions, enhancing emotional regulation.

Scientific studies and expert insights provided compelling evidence for the effectiveness of mental health exercises. The concept of brain reshaping and plasticity highlighted the tangible changes occurring within our brains as a result of these practices. Ultimately, we discovered that mental health exercises contribute to better overall well-being by fostering resilience and emotional balance.

Chapter 9 - The Connection Between Mind and Body

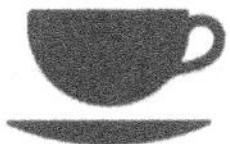

The mind-body connection is a crucial aspect of emotional well-being. In this section, we elucidate the profound link between our mental and physical health. We delve into the impact of exercise, nutrition, and sleep on our emotional well-being. Practical tips and evidence-based strategies for maintaining a holistic and healthy lifestyle are provided.

The mind-body connection is a fundamental concept in understanding human well-being. It refers to the intricate relationship between our mental and physical health, demonstrating how they influence and depend on each other. This connection is not merely a theoretical concept; it has a profound impact on our daily lives and emotional well-being. In this comprehensive exploration, we will delve into the intricacies of the mind-body connection, focusing on the role of exercise, nutrition, and sleep in maintaining emotional well-being. Throughout this discussion, we will provide practical tips and evidence-based strategies to help individuals foster a holistic and healthy lifestyle.

I. Understanding the Mind-Body Connection

1.1. The Historical Perspective

The concept of the mind-body connection has deep historical roots, with various philosophical, medical, and cultural perspectives shaping our understanding. Ancient civilizations, such as the Greeks and Egyptians, recognized this connection, attributing emotional and physical ailments to a harmonious or discordant balance between the mind and body. Similarly, Eastern traditions, like Ayurveda and

Traditional Chinese Medicine, emphasized the interdependence of mental and physical health.

1.2. Modern Scientific Perspective

In the modern era, scientific research has provided substantial evidence supporting the existence of the mind-body connection. Neuroscientific studies reveal the intricate networks and pathways that link the brain and the body, demonstrating that our thoughts and emotions can profoundly influence physiological processes. Furthermore, psychological research highlights how emotional well-being impacts mental health and vice versa.

1.3. The Stress Response

One of the clearest examples of the mind-body connection is the body's stress response. When we encounter stress, whether from a psychological source (e.g., work-related pressure) or a physical one (e.g., an injury), our body releases stress hormones like cortisol. This physiological response can affect our mood, sleep, and overall emotional well-being. Chronic stress, in particular, has been linked to various mental health issues, including anxiety and depression.

II. The Role of Exercise in Emotional Well-being

2.1. Exercise and Brain Health

Physical activity has a profound impact on the brain. When we exercise, our brain releases neurotransmitters like endorphins and serotonin, which are known to improve mood and reduce stress. Regular exercise has been linked to enhanced cognitive function, improved memory, and a reduced risk of neurodegenerative diseases.

2.2. Stress Reduction

Exercise serves as a powerful tool for stress reduction. It helps dissipate the physical tension associated with stress and can also modulate the body's stress response by lowering cortisol levels. Engaging in physical activities like yoga, meditation, or aerobic exercises has been shown to alleviate symptoms of anxiety and depression.

2.3. The Role of Endorphins

Endorphins, often referred to as "feel-good" hormones, are released during exercise. These natural painkillers not only reduce discomfort but also generate a sense of well-being and happiness. Understanding the connection between endorphin release and exercise can motivate individuals to incorporate physical activity into their daily routines.

2.4. Long-term Mental Health Benefits

Regular exercise has long-term mental health benefits. It can reduce the risk of developing mood disorders, such as depression and anxiety, and can be an effective part of their treatment. Moreover, it enhances self-esteem and self-confidence, contributing to overall emotional well-being.

2.5. Practical Tips for Incorporating Exercise

To harness the emotional benefits of exercise, individuals can consider various activities that suit their preferences and lifestyles. Some practical tips include setting achievable fitness goals, finding enjoyable forms of exercise, and establishing a consistent routine.

III. Nutrition and Emotional Well-being

3.1. The Gut-Brain Connection

Emerging research has unveiled the intricate relationship between the gut and the brain, often referred to as the "gut-brain axis." The gut contains a complex ecosystem of microorganisms known as the gut microbiota, which play a crucial role in regulating mood and emotions. The composition of the gut microbiota can be influenced by diet and, in turn, affect emotional well-being.

3.2. Nutrient Influence on Mood

Certain nutrients have been shown to influence mood and emotional well-being. For example, omega-3 fatty acids, found in fatty fish and flaxseeds, have anti-inflammatory properties and may help reduce symptoms of depression. Similarly, foods rich in antioxidants, like fruits and vegetables, can protect against oxidative stress, which is linked to mood disorders.

3.3. The Role of Sugar and Processed Foods

Excessive consumption of sugar and highly processed foods has been associated with mood swings, energy crashes, and increased risk of depression. These foods can lead to rapid spikes and crashes in blood sugar levels, affecting mood stability. Reducing the intake of such foods is essential for maintaining emotional well-being.

3.4. The Impact of Hydration

Dehydration can lead to cognitive deficits, fatigue, and mood disturbances. Staying adequately hydrated is a simple yet often overlooked aspect of nutrition that can significantly impact mental clarity and emotional balance.

3.5. Mindful Eating

Practicing mindful eating involves paying full attention to the sensory experience of eating. This approach can help individuals make healthier food choices, enjoy their meals more, and maintain a balanced relationship with food, all of which contribute to emotional well-being.

IV. The Crucial Role of Sleep in Emotional Well-being

4.1. Sleep and Brain Function

Sleep is a fundamental physiological process that plays a vital role in maintaining cognitive and emotional well-being. During sleep, the brain undergoes critical processes like memory consolidation and emotional regulation. Lack of sleep can impair these functions, leading to mood disturbances.

4.2. Sleep and Stress Reduction

A good night's sleep is essential for stress reduction. Sleep deprivation increases the body's stress response, elevating cortisol levels. Chronic sleep problems can contribute to chronic stress and exacerbate emotional disorders.

4.3. The Circadian Rhythm

Our body's internal clock, known as the circadian rhythm, regulates the sleep-wake cycle. Disruptions to this rhythm, such as irregular sleep patterns or exposure to artificial light at night, can negatively affect emotional well-being. Maintaining a consistent sleep schedule and creating a sleep-conducive environment are crucial for mental health.

4.4. Sleep Disorders and Mental Health

Various sleep disorders, such as insomnia and sleep apnea, are closely linked to mental health issues. Treating these sleep disorders can lead to significant improvements in emotional well-being.

4.5. Tips for Better Sleep

To optimize sleep quality and emotional well-being, individuals can adopt healthy sleep habits, also known as sleep hygiene. These include establishing a bedtime routine, creating a comfortable sleep environment, and limiting exposure to screens before bedtime.

V. Holistic Strategies for Emotional Well-being

5.1. The Synergy of Exercise, Nutrition, and Sleep

To achieve optimal emotional well-being, it is essential to recognize the synergy between exercise, nutrition, and sleep. A holistic approach that incorporates all three elements can have a more significant impact on mental health than focusing on each in isolation.

5.2. Stress Management Techniques

Incorporating stress management techniques, such as mindfulness meditation, deep breathing exercises, or progressive muscle relaxation, can further enhance emotional well-being. These practices help individuals cope with stress and promote mental clarity.

5.3. Social Connection and Emotional Support

Maintaining strong social connections and seeking emotional support from friends, family, or support groups is critical

Chapter 10 - Benefits Beyond Measure

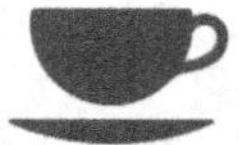

Building upon the scientific foundations laid in the previous sections, we proceed to outline the multifaceted benefits of engaging in mental health exercises. We illustrate how these exercises lead to stress reduction, heightened resilience, improved relationships, and increased productivity. By understanding the comprehensive advantages, readers gain a deeper appreciation for the transformative potential of these exercises.

In today's fast-paced and increasingly complex world, the importance of mental health has never been more evident. Mental health exercises, encompassing a wide range of practices and strategies, offer individuals the means to nurture their emotional well-being and resilience. Building upon the scientific foundations of the mind-body connection discussed previously, this comprehensive exploration aims to elucidate the multifaceted benefits of engaging in mental health exercises. By delving into the realms of stress reduction, heightened resilience, improved relationships, and increased productivity, readers will gain a profound appreciation for the transformative potential of these exercises.

I. Stress Reduction: The Gateway to Emotional Balance

1.1. Understanding Stress

Stress is an inherent part of life, but excessive or chronic stress can have detrimental effects on both mental and physical health. Mental health exercises provide a means to mitigate the impact of stress and enhance emotional well-being.

1.2. Mindfulness Meditation

Mindfulness meditation is a powerful mental health exercise that involves paying non-judgmental attention to the present moment. Numerous studies have shown that regular mindfulness practice can reduce stress levels, lower cortisol (a stress hormone) production, and improve overall emotional well-being.

1.3. Breathing Techniques

Breathing exercises, such as deep diaphragmatic breathing or the 4-7-8 technique, help activate the body's relaxation response. These exercises can be easily integrated into daily routines, providing quick and effective stress relief.

1.4. Progressive Muscle Relaxation

Progressive muscle relaxation involves systematically tensing and then relaxing different muscle groups. This technique can help release physical tension and alleviate the physical symptoms of stress, such as headaches and muscle aches.

1.5. Art Therapy and Creative Expression

Engaging in creative activities like painting, drawing, or writing can serve as a form of emotional release and stress reduction. Creative expression allows individuals to channel their emotions and thoughts into a tangible form, promoting self-awareness and emotional balance.

II. Heightened Resilience: Building Emotional Strength

2.1. Resilience Defined

Resilience is the ability to bounce back from adversity and maintain emotional well-being in the face of life's challenges. Mental health exercises play a pivotal role in building and enhancing resilience.

2.2. Cognitive Behavioral Therapy (CBT)

CBT is a widely recognized therapeutic approach that helps individuals identify and challenge negative thought patterns and beliefs. By learning to reframe their thinking, individuals can develop a more resilient mindset.

2.3. Gratitude Practice

Cultivating gratitude involves focusing on the positive aspects of life and acknowledging one's blessings. Regular gratitude practice has been shown to enhance resilience by shifting focus away from negative experiences and promoting a more optimistic outlook.

2.4. Journaling and Self-Reflection

Keeping a journal allows individuals to explore their thoughts and emotions, providing a valuable tool for self-reflection and personal growth. Journaling can help individuals process challenging experiences and develop resilience through self-awareness.

2.5. Emotional Intelligence (EQ)

Emotional intelligence, the ability to recognize, understand, and manage emotions, is a key component of resilience. Mental health exercises that enhance emotional awareness and regulation can improve an individual's ability to navigate difficult situations.

III. Improved Relationships: The Heart of Emotional Well-being

3.1. The Role of Relationships

Quality relationships are integral to emotional well-being. Mental health exercises can enhance interpersonal skills, communication, and empathy, leading to healthier and more fulfilling relationships.

3.2. Empathy and Compassion Training

Empathy and compassion are crucial for building strong connections with others. Exercises that cultivate empathy and compassion, such as loving-kindness meditation, can improve the quality of relationships by fostering understanding and support.

3.3. Effective Communication

Effective communication is the cornerstone of healthy relationships. Mental health exercises that focus on active listening, assertiveness, and conflict resolution can help individuals express themselves more clearly and connect on a deeper level with others.

3.4. Building Trust

Trust is a vital component of any relationship, and mental health exercises can help individuals rebuild trust after it has been damaged. These exercises often involve self-reflection, forgiveness, and empathy toward oneself and others.

3.5. Family and Couples Therapy

In situations where relationships are strained or facing challenges, family and couples therapy can be an effective form of mental health exercise. These therapeutic interventions provide a structured environment for addressing issues and improving relationship dynamics.

IV. Increased Productivity: Mindfulness in Action

4.1. Productivity and Mental Health

Mental health exercises are not limited to reducing stress or improving relationships; they can also significantly impact productivity. When individuals are emotionally balanced and mentally resilient, they are better equipped to excel in their professional endeavors.

4.2. Mindful Productivity

Mindfulness extends beyond stress reduction; it can be harnessed to enhance productivity. By practicing mindfulness in the workplace, individuals can improve their focus, decision-making, and time management skills.

4.3. Stress Management for Work

Stress is a common contributor to reduced productivity at work. Mental health exercises that address workplace stress, such as setting boundaries, prioritizing tasks, and practicing relaxation techniques, can help individuals maintain peak performance.

4.4. Creativity and Innovation

Enhanced emotional well-being can also stimulate creativity and innovation. Mental health exercises that encourage thinking outside the box and embracing change can lead to breakthroughs and increased productivity in various fields.

4.5. Work-Life Balance

Balancing work and personal life is essential for overall well-being and productivity. Mental health exercises that promote work-life balance, such as time management and boundary-setting, can lead to increased job satisfaction and professional success.

V. Conclusion: A Life Enriched Through Mental Health Exercises

5.1. The Transformative Potential

The benefits of mental health exercises extend far beyond stress reduction. They encompass heightened resilience, improved relationships, and increased productivity. By engaging in these exercises, individuals can experience profound personal growth and enrichment.

5.2. The Holistic Approach

To fully embrace the advantages of mental health exercises, it is crucial to adopt a holistic approach. This involves integrating various exercises and strategies into daily life, recognizing that emotional well-being is interconnected with physical health, relationships, and professional success.

5.3. The Ongoing Journey

Embracing mental health exercises is not a one-time endeavor but an ongoing journey. Just as physical exercise requires consistency to maintain physical health, mental health exercises require dedication and practice to sustain emotional well-being.

The multifaceted benefits of mental health exercises are truly beyond measure. These exercises serve as tools for navigating the complexities of life, fostering emotional balance, and enriching our relationships and productivity. By understanding and embracing the transformative potential of these exercises, individuals can embark on a journey towards a more fulfilling and emotionally resilient life.

Chapter 11 - Overcoming Common Barriers

Engaging in mental health exercises can be a challenge, with common barriers like time constraints and self-doubt often standing in the way. In this section, we address these hurdles head-on, offering practical strategies and insights to empower readers to overcome obstacles. By acknowledging and navigating these barriers, individuals can better integrate mental health exercises into their daily routines.

Engaging in mental health exercises is a vital aspect of maintaining emotional well-being and resilience. However, the journey to incorporating these exercises into daily life is often met with various challenges and barriers. This comprehensive exploration aims to address these hurdles head-on and provide practical strategies and insights to empower readers to overcome obstacles. By acknowledging and navigating these common barriers, individuals can better integrate mental health exercises into their daily routines, ultimately fostering a more balanced and emotionally resilient life.

I. The Time Constraint Dilemma

1.1. The Importance of Prioritizing Mental Health

In today's fast-paced world, time is a precious resource, and individuals often struggle to allocate it to activities that promote mental health. To overcome this common barrier, it's essential to recognize the significance of prioritizing mental health exercises.

1.2. The Myth of Time Scarcity

Many people believe they lack the time for mental health exercises due to busy schedules. However, it's crucial to challenge the myth of time scarcity and acknowledge that making time for mental health is an investment in overall well-being.

1.3. Strategies for Time Management

Effective time management is key to overcoming the time constraint barrier. Techniques such as setting clear priorities, creating a daily schedule, and eliminating time-wasting activities can help individuals carve out time for mental health exercises.

1.4. Incorporating Mental Health into Daily Routines

Instead of viewing mental health exercises as separate tasks, individuals can integrate them into existing daily routines. This approach can make these exercises more accessible and sustainable.

1.5. Short, Effective Practices

Not all mental health exercises require extended periods of time. Short, focused practices like five-minute mindfulness sessions or quick journaling exercises can provide significant benefits without demanding excessive time commitments.

II. Self-Doubt and Resistance

2.1. The Inner Critic

Self-doubt and resistance often stem from the inner critic, that nagging voice that tells us we're not good enough or capable of change. Overcoming this barrier requires understanding and managing our inner critic.

2.2. Cultivating Self-Compassion

Self-compassion is the antidote to self-doubt. It involves treating ourselves with the same kindness and understanding that we would offer a friend. By nurturing self-compassion, individuals can silence their inner critics and approach mental health exercises with greater self-assurance.

2.3. Overcoming Perfectionism

Perfectionism is a common obstacle that can prevent individuals from engaging in mental health exercises.

Recognizing that perfection is not the goal and that progress, no matter how small, is valuable, can help individuals overcome this barrier.

2.4. The Power of Self-Reflection

Engaging in self-reflection allows individuals to explore their doubts and resistance to mental health exercises. Through journaling or conversations with a therapist or coach, individuals can gain insights into the root causes of their self-doubt and develop strategies to overcome it.

2.5. Embracing Small Steps

Overcoming self-doubt often requires taking small, manageable steps toward engaging in mental health exercises. Setting achievable goals and acknowledging successes, no matter how minor, can build confidence and motivation.

III. Lack of Motivation and Consistency

3.1. The Motivation Rollercoaster

Motivation can be elusive, and many individuals struggle to maintain consistency in their mental health exercise routines. Understanding the nature of motivation and developing strategies to sustain it is essential.

3.2. Setting Meaningful Goals

Motivation is closely tied to the perceived value of a task. By setting meaningful, personally relevant goals for mental health exercises, individuals can increase their intrinsic motivation to engage in these activities regularly.

3.3. Creating a Supportive Environment

The environment in which mental health exercises take place can significantly impact motivation and consistency. Creating a supportive and inviting space for these activities can make them more appealing and accessible.

3.4. Accountability and Tracking Progress

Accountability partners or tracking progress through journaling can help individuals stay motivated and consistent. Sharing their goals and progress with others can provide encouragement and a sense of responsibility.

3.5. The Role of Routine

Incorporating mental health exercises into a daily or weekly routine can foster consistency. When these exercises become habitual, individuals are less likely to skip them due to lack of motivation.

IV. Fear of Vulnerability

4.1. The Fear of Being Vulnerable

Engaging in mental health exercises often requires individuals to confront their emotions, thoughts, and vulnerabilities. The fear of being vulnerable can be a significant barrier, as it involves stepping outside one's comfort zone.

4.2. The Benefits of Vulnerability

It's essential to recognize that vulnerability is not a weakness but a source of strength. Being open and honest about one's emotions and challenges can lead to personal growth, deeper connections with others, and increased self-acceptance.

4.3. Building Trust

Overcoming the fear of vulnerability often involves building trust, both in oneself and in the process of mental health exercises. Trusting that these activities are safe and beneficial is a crucial step toward engagement.

4.4. Seeking Support and Guidance

In cases where the fear of vulnerability is particularly daunting, seeking support from a therapist, counselor, or support group can provide a safe space to explore and address vulnerabilities.

4.5. Self-Compassion and Self-Acceptance

Practicing self-compassion and self-acceptance can help individuals navigate their vulnerabilities with greater ease. Recognizing that everyone has vulnerabilities and that they do not diminish one's worth is a powerful mindset shift.

V. The Influence of External Factors

5.1. External Barriers

External factors such as financial constraints, lack of access to resources, or unsupportive environments can hinder individuals from engaging in mental health exercises. Addressing these external barriers is crucial for empowerment.

5.2. Resourcefulness and Adaptability

Developing resourcefulness and adaptability is key to overcoming external barriers. Individuals can explore low-cost or free resources, seek community support, and adapt mental health exercises to fit their unique circumstances.

5.3. Advocating for Change

In situations where external barriers are systemic or widespread, individuals can advocate for change at a broader level. By raising awareness and advocating for improved access to mental health resources, individuals can contribute to positive change in their communities.

5.4. Building a Support Network

Creating a support network of friends, family, or like-minded individuals who share similar goals can help individuals overcome external barriers. Collaborative efforts can provide motivation and practical solutions to common challenges.

Overcoming common barriers to mental health exercises is an empowering journey that requires self-awareness, self-compassion, and determination. By prioritizing mental health, challenging self-doubt, sustaining motivation, embracing vulnerability, and addressing external factors, individuals can build emotional resilience and lead more balanced and fulfilling lives. Ultimately, the ability to overcome these barriers is a testament to the transformative potential of mental health exercises, allowing individuals to thrive in the face of life's challenges.

Chapter 12 - Your Journey Begins: Practical Mental Health Exercises

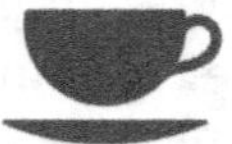

The heart of the book unfolds in this section, where we introduce a diverse array of practical mental health exercises. Each exercise is meticulously explained, providing step-by-step guidance on how to incorporate them into one's daily life. These exercises encompass mindfulness practices, journaling prompts, relaxation techniques, and gratitude exercises, among others. Real-life testimonials from individuals who have experienced transformation through these exercises serve as a source of inspiration.

Mindfulness practices are the cornerstone of this journey. They are simple yet profound techniques that can help you cultivate awareness, reduce stress, and improve your overall sense of well-being. Through mindfulness, you will learn to be fully present in each moment, to observe your thoughts and feelings without judgment, and to create space for a more peaceful mind.

The Power of Mindfulness

In a world characterized by constant distractions, relentless schedules, and the ever-present digital buzz, finding moments of peace and clarity can seem like an elusive dream. Yet, within the realm of mindfulness, you'll uncover the invaluable tools to help you reclaim your inner calm, cultivate profound awareness, and enhance your overall well-being.

Mindfulness Practices: Your Foundation for Inner Peace

Mindfulness practices serve as the cornerstone of your journey towards improved mental health. These techniques may appear deceptively simple, but their impact is nothing short of profound. At their core, mindfulness exercises encourage you to engage with the present moment, free from the shackles of the past or the worries of the future. Through mindfulness, you'll embark on a path towards self-discovery, emotional regulation, and a more tranquil existence.

The Essence of Mindfulness: Being Fully Present

Central to mindfulness is the art of being fully present. It is a state of being in which you immerse yourself wholeheartedly in whatever you are doing or experiencing. When you eat, you truly taste and savor your food. When you walk, you feel the earth beneath your feet and the breeze on your skin. When you engage in conversation, you listen with unwavering attention.

Observing Without Judgment

A fundamental aspect of mindfulness is the practice of observing your thoughts, emotions, and sensations without judgment. Imagine your mind as a vast sky, and your thoughts and feelings as passing clouds. Instead of getting caught up in the storms or clinging to the pleasant clouds, you learn to watch them come and go. This non-judgmental observation creates a sense of detachment from your thoughts and emotions, allowing you to respond to life's challenges with greater clarity and equanimity.

Creating Space for Inner Peace

As you embrace mindfulness, you'll gradually carve out a serene sanctuary within your mind a space where the noise of anxiety, worry, and stress fades into the background. This inner oasis becomes a refuge you can retreat to whenever the demands of life become overwhelming.

Exploring Mindfulness Exercises: Your Toolkit for Well-Being

In the pages ahead, we'll embark on a journey through various mindfulness exercises, each designed to offer you a unique path towards tranquility and self-awareness. Some of these exercises may be familiar, while others might be new territory. Regardless of your prior experience, we'll provide clear and accessible guidance for every step of the way.

Mindful Breathing: Discover the art of anchoring your awareness in the rhythmic rise and fall of your breath. This foundational practice forms the bedrock of mindfulness and can be integrated seamlessly into your daily routine.

Body Scans: Explore the landscape of your own body through guided body scan meditations. These exercises facilitate the release of tension and promote a profound sense of bodily awareness.

Mindful Eating: Transform your relationship with food by savoring each bite and engaging all your senses during meals. Mindful eating not only nourishes your body but also deepens your connection to the act of eating.

Walking Meditation: Turn your daily stroll into a mindfulness practice. Learn how to take each step with intention, grounding yourself in the present moment as you move through the world.

Mindful Listening: Elevate your communication skills by truly listening to others with undivided attention. Mindful listening fosters more meaningful connections and enhances your understanding of those around you.

Integration into Your Daily Life

Practicality is key when it comes to mindfulness. We'll offer practical tips on seamlessly integrating these exercises into your daily routine. From finding the right time to practice to creating dedicated spaces for mindfulness, we'll help you make mindfulness a part of your life, rather than just a sporadic endeavor.

Navigating Life's Challenges with Equanimity

As you go deeper into mindfulness practices, you'll come to understand that they are not merely tools for stress reduction, but profound instruments for navigating life's ups and downs. With mindfulness as your guide, you'll develop the ability to respond to adversity with grace, make decisions from a place of clarity, and find solace in the midst of chaos.

The journey of mindfulness is a transformative one, leading you to a place of heightened awareness, inner peace, and greater resilience. So, let's embark on this voyage together, one mindful breath at a time, as we explore the limitless potential of your own mind.

Sarah's story is a compelling testament to the transformative power of mindfulness in the realm of mental well-being. As a corporate executive grappling with chronic stress and anxiety, she embarked on a profound journey of self-discovery and healing, and through mindfulness exercises, she found her lifeline to inner peace and resilience.

The Demands of Corporate Life

Corporate life can be fast-paced and demanding, and for Sarah, it became a constant source of stress and anxiety. The pressures of managing teams, meeting deadlines, and navigating the competitive landscape took a toll on her mental and emotional well-being.

The Turning Point

One day, Sarah reached a breaking point. The incessant stress had begun to affect her physical health, and she realized that something had to change. In her search for relief, she stumbled upon mindfulness through an article in a health magazine.

Discovering Mindfulness

Sarah began exploring mindfulness through guided meditation apps and online resources. Mindfulness, she learned, was the practice of being fully present in the moment, of observing thoughts and feelings without judgment, and of cultivating self-awareness.

Mindfulness as a Lifeline

The impact of mindfulness on Sarah's life was profound. She found that mindfulness exercises provided her with a lifeline to navigate the turbulent waters of her mind. Mindfulness helped her break free from the relentless cycle of stress and anxiety by allowing her to detach from her worries and rumination.

Managing Stress and Anxiety

Through mindfulness, Sarah learned to manage her stress and anxiety effectively. She discovered that by grounding herself in the present moment, she could observe her anxious thoughts without becoming entangled in them. Mindfulness breathing exercises became her go-to technique for calming her racing mind and soothing her frazzled nerves.

Embracing Self-Compassion

A crucial aspect of Sarah's mindfulness journey was the cultivation of self-compassion. She realized that, as a corporate executive, she had often been too hard on herself, setting impossibly high standards. Mindfulness taught her to treat herself with kindness and understanding, allowing her to let go of perfectionism and self-criticism.

Enhancing Emotional Regulation

Mindfulness exercises also played a pivotal role in enhancing Sarah's emotional regulation. By regularly practicing mindfulness, she became more attuned to her emotions as they arose. This heightened awareness allowed her to respond to situations with greater emotional intelligence, leading to more harmonious relationships at work and at home.

A Deeper Sense of Well-Being

Over time, Sarah's mindfulness practice led to a deeper sense of well-being. She experienced increased moments of joy, gratitude, and contentment in her daily life. The persistent undercurrent of anxiety that had accompanied her for years began to recede, replaced by a sense of calm and equanimity.

Sharing the Gift of Mindfulness

As Sarah continued her mindfulness journey, she felt compelled to share this gift with others. She introduced mindfulness practices in her workplace, leading meditation sessions for her colleagues during lunch breaks. Witnessing the positive impact, it had on their well-being further reinforced her commitment to mindfulness.

The Ongoing Path of Mindfulness

Sarah's journey is ongoing, a reminder that mindfulness is not a destination but a continuous practice. It's a journey of self-discovery, self-compassion, and self-mastery. Through mindfulness, Sarah discovered the power to reclaim her mental well-being and found a profound sense of peace amidst life's challenges.

Sarah's story is a testament to the transformative potential of mindfulness, offering hope to those who battle stress and anxiety. Her journey illustrates that, no matter how demanding or overwhelming life may become, the practice of mindfulness can provide solace, resilience, and a path to mental well-being. Through mindfulness exercises, Sarah found her lifeline, and in doing so, she discovered the profound gift of inner peace.

Journaling for Self-Discovery

In the age of digital communication and constant busyness, the simple act of putting pen to paper holds a unique power. It is a gateway to the inner recesses of your mind, a channel through which your thoughts and emotions flow freely onto the pages of a journal. Welcome to the world of journaling, a profound tool for self-reflection and self-discovery.

The Untapped Potential of Journaling

At first glance, journaling may seem like an ordinary practice a mundane exercise in recording daily events or jotting down thoughts. However, beneath its unassuming surface lies a transformative force. Journaling is a sanctuary where you can explore the depths of your consciousness, untangle the intricacies of your emotions, and unearth the buried treasures of self-awareness.

The Journal as Your Confidant

Think of your journal as a trusted confidant, a non-judgmental listener who eagerly awaits your words. It is a safe space where you can be unapologetically yourself, express your innermost thoughts, and release the burdens that weigh on your heart. Through this act of self-expression, you embark on a journey of self-discovery and healing.

Journaling Prompts: The Catalysts of Transformation

In this section, we will introduce you to a collection of journaling prompts meticulously designed to guide you on your voyage of self-discovery. These prompts are more than just words; they are keys that unlock the doors to your inner world. Whether you find yourself grappling with difficult emotions, seeking clarity in your life's path, or simply wishing to document your daily thoughts, these prompts will serve as your companions on this introspective journey.

Getting Started: Setting Up Your Journaling Routine

Before we dive into the prompts, let's establish the foundations of a productive journaling practice. Here are some essential steps to get you started:

1. Choose Your Journal: Select a journal that resonates with you. Whether it's a sleek leather-bound book or a digital note-taking app, find a medium that feels comfortable and inviting.

2. Find Your Time: Identify a time in your day when you can commit to journaling. It could be in the morning to set intentions for the day, in the evening to reflect on your experiences, or any other time that suits your routine.

3. Create a Ritual: Establish a ritual around your journaling practice. Light a candle, sip a cup of tea, or play soft music whatever helps you transition into a reflective state of mind.

4. Embrace Consistency: Consistency is key. Aim to journal regularly, whether it's daily, weekly, or at any frequency that suits your lifestyle.

5. Set an Intention: Before you begin, set an intention for your journaling session. What do you hope to explore or gain insight into today? Setting an intention gives your journaling purpose and direction.

The Power of Prompts: A Journey Within

Now, let's go into the heart of journaling exploring the world within you through carefully crafted prompts. Here is a taste of what you can expect:

1. Gratitude Journaling: Begin your journaling journey by acknowledging the blessings in your life. Write down three

things you are grateful for today and reflect on why they bring you joy.

2. Emotion Exploration: Dive deep into your emotional landscape. Describe a recent emotional experience in detail. What triggered it? How did it manifest in your body and mind? What did you learn from it?

3. Life Vision: Envision your ideal life five years from now. Describe it in vivid detail your career, relationships, hobbies, and personal growth. What steps can you take today to align with this vision?

4. Self-Compassion: Write a letter to yourself as if you were your own best friend. Offer words of kindness, encouragement, and support. What would you say to uplift your spirits?

5. Reflect on Challenges: Explore a recent challenge or adversity you've faced. How did you handle it? What did you learn from the experience? How can you grow from it?

6. Daily Reflection: At the end of each day, reflect on your experiences and emotions. What were the highlights and low points of your day? How did you respond to them? What insights can you carry forward?

The Journey Unfolds

Through these journaling prompts and the act of putting your thoughts and emotions into words, you will gradually gain deeper insights into yourself, your values, and your goals. You'll discover the threads that connect your past, present, and future, as well as the patterns that shape your thoughts and behaviors.

Journaling is not just about documenting your life; it's about actively participating in your own growth and self-discovery. As you embark on this journaling journey, remember that it is a process, not a destination. With each entry, you take a step closer to understanding yourself and finding clarity amidst life's complexities.

So, let your journal be your faithful companion on this quest for self-discovery. Embrace the power of your words, and let them illuminate the path to a more profound understanding of yourself and the world around you.

Mark's journey is a compelling testament to the transformative power of journaling in the realm of self-discovery and personal growth. As a college student grappling with identity and self-esteem issues, he embarked on a journey of profound introspection and healing, and through journaling, he found the compass to navigate the complexities of his inner world.

The Struggles of College Life

College life can be both exciting and overwhelming, and for Mark, it was a time marked by uncertainty and self-doubt. He was searching for his identity and purpose, often feeling lost in a sea of academic pressures and social expectations.

The Discovery of Journaling

One day, while seeking solace in a local bookstore, Mark stumbled upon a blank journal. This simple act of purchasing a journal marked the beginning of a profound transformation. Initially, he had no specific purpose for this journal, but it soon became a sanctuary for his thoughts, emotions, and innermost fears.

The Healing Power of Expression

Mark discovered that journaling provided a safe and non-judgmental space to express his thoughts and feelings. The act of writing allowed him to externalize the chaos within, making it more manageable. He found that the simple act of putting words on paper could be cathartic, releasing the emotional weight that had burdened him for so long.

Self-Reflection and Self-Discovery

As he continued to journal, Mark started to notice patterns in his thoughts and emotions. He began to ask himself fundamental questions about his desires, values, and dreams. This process of self-reflection opened a door to self-discovery. Through journaling, he unearthed his passions and strengths, gradually piecing together a clearer image of who he was and what he aspired to be.

Challenging Negative Self-Talk

Mark was no stranger to the corrosive effects of negative self-talk. He realized that journaling could be a powerful tool in challenging and reframing these self-limiting beliefs. He used his journal to identify the roots of his self-esteem issues and to develop more positive and affirming self-talk.

Goal Setting and Personal Growth

With his journal as a guide, Mark began to set clear goals for personal growth. He wrote down aspirations, both short-term and long-term, and outlined the steps he needed to take to achieve them. This proactive approach empowered him to move beyond the inertia that had held him back.

A Compass for Life's Journey

Mark's journal became a compass for navigating the complexities of his life. It served as a record of his progress, a source of inspiration during challenging times, and a reminder of the path he had chosen. Through journaling, he discovered a sense of purpose and direction that had eluded him before.

Sharing His Journey

Over time, Mark recognized that his journaling journey was not only a deeply personal one but also a story that could inspire and help others. He began to share his experiences through blog posts and public speaking engagements, aiming to encourage others to embark on their own journeys of self-discovery through journaling.

The Ongoing Process of Growth

Mark's journey is a continual one, a reminder that self-discovery and personal growth are lifelong processes. His journal remains a trusted companion on this path, a space where he records not only his successes but also his setbacks and lessons learned.

Mark's story illustrates how journaling can be a powerful tool for self-discovery and personal growth. It's a testament to the fact that, no matter where we are on our life's journey, we have the power to introspect, heal, and grow. Through journaling, Mark found his compass, and in doing so, he discovered a profound sense of self-worth and direction. His journey serves as an inspiration to others to embark on their own voyage of self-discovery through the pages of a journal.

Finding Serenity Through Relaxation Techniques

In the ceaseless whirlwind of our modern lives, finding moments of serenity and calm may seem like an elusive dream. The demands of work, the cacophony of daily responsibilities, and the constant digital bombardment can leave us feeling frazzled and disconnected from our inner peace. However, in this section, we will unlock the secret to tranquility through a range of relaxation techniques.

The Importance of Relaxation in Mental Well-being

Before we dive into these techniques, it's essential to recognize the significance of relaxation in the context of mental well-being. In a world where stress and anxiety often take center stage, relaxation serves as a vital counterbalance. It is not a luxury but a necessity for maintaining mental and emotional equilibrium.

Exploring Relaxation Techniques: Your Path to Inner Peace

This section is your gateway to a world of relaxation techniques, each carefully selected to help you reduce anxiety, lower stress levels, and cultivate a profound sense of inner peace. These practices are accessible, adaptable, and can be seamlessly woven into the fabric of your daily life.

Progressive Muscle Relaxation

Progressive muscle relaxation is a technique that focuses on systematically tensing and then relaxing different muscle groups in your body. By doing so, you release physical tension, which, in turn, helps ease emotional stress.

Instructions:

Find a quiet and comfortable space.

Start with your toes and work your way up through your body, tensing each muscle group for a few seconds and then releasing.

Pay close attention to the sensations of tension and relaxation in each muscle.

Breathe deeply and calmly as you proceed.

Progressive muscle relaxation can be particularly effective when you're feeling physically tense or after a stressful day.

Deep Breathing Exercises

Deep breathing exercises are simple yet potent tools for calming the mind and relaxing the body. They are easily accessible and can be practiced virtually anywhere.

Instructions:

Find a quiet space, sit or lie down in a comfortable position.

Inhale deeply through your nose for a count of four.

Hold your breath for a count of four.

Exhale slowly and completely through your mouth for a count of six.

Repeat this cycle several times, focusing on your breath and the rhythm of your inhales and exhales.

Deep breathing exercises can be practiced during moments of stress, before important meetings, or whenever you need to regain composure and clarity.

Guided Imagery

Guided imagery is a practice that involves using your imagination to create a mental image that promotes relaxation and reduces stress. It's like taking a mental vacation to a serene and calming place.

Instructions:

Find a quiet, comfortable space.

Close your eyes and take a few deep breaths to center yourself.

Imagine a peaceful and soothing place, such as a beach, forest, or meadow.

Engage all your senses as you immerse yourself in this mental landscape. Feel the warmth of the sun, hear the rustling of leaves, and smell the fragrant flowers.

Spend a few minutes in this calming mental space, allowing yourself to relax and let go of stress.

Guided imagery can transport you to a place of tranquility and serve as a mental escape from the demands of daily life.

Integration into Daily Life

Relaxation techniques are most effective when integrated into your daily routine. Consider the following tips for seamless incorporation:

Set aside time: Dedicate a specific time each day for relaxation, even if it's just a few minutes.

Use triggers: Connect relaxation practices to existing routines, like deep breathing during your morning coffee or progressive muscle relaxation before bedtime.

Create a calming environment: Make your relaxation space inviting with soothing colors, comfortable cushions, and soft lighting.

By incorporating these techniques into your life, you will create a sanctuary of tranquility amidst the chaos, providing you with the tools to navigate life's challenges with greater ease and a profound sense of inner peace. Relaxation is not a luxury but a necessity for your mental well-being, and it is within your reach, waiting to be embraced.

Cultivating Gratitude

In a world often overshadowed by the clamor of desires and the pursuit of more, cultivating gratitude emerges as a profound antidote. It is the art of shifting one's gaze from the void of lack to the richness of abundance, from discontentment to contentment. In this section, we embark on a journey to explore the transformative power of gratitude.

The Essence of Gratitude

Gratitude is more than a mere polite expression of thanks; it is a fundamental shift in perspective. It invites us to recognize the beauty and blessings in our lives, no matter how small or seemingly insignificant. It is the practice of acknowledging the gifts that surround us daily, from the warmth of the sun on our skin to the love of family and friends.

The Power of a Grateful Mindset

A grateful mindset is not just about feeling good; it has a profound impact on our mental and emotional well-being. It reduces stress, increases resilience, and enhances overall life satisfaction. When we train our minds to focus on the positive aspects of life, we naturally become more attuned to joy and contentment.

Gratitude Exercises: Nurturing a Grateful Heart

This section introduces a variety of gratitude exercises that serve as tools to develop and nurture a grateful mindset. These exercises are simple yet potent, helping you shift your focus towards the abundance that surrounds you.

1. Gratitude Journaling

Instructions:

Set aside a dedicated journal for your gratitude practice.

Each day, write down three things you are grateful for.

Reflect on why these things bring you joy and how they enrich your life.

Gratitude journaling is a powerful daily practice that reminds you of the blessings, both big and small, that grace your life. It helps you cultivate a habit of acknowledging and appreciating the positive aspects of each day.

2. Gratitude in Relationships

Instructions:

Take a moment to express gratitude to someone in your life.

Write a heartfelt note, send a text, or simply tell them face-to-face.

Be specific about what you appreciate about them and how they have made a difference in your life.

Practicing gratitude in relationships strengthens bonds, fosters connection, and spreads positivity. It reminds us of the value of the people who enrich our lives and encourages us to express our appreciation.

3. Savoring the Small Joys

Instructions:

Take a pause during your day to savor a small joy.

It could be a moment of sunshine, the taste of your favorite food, or the laughter of a loved one.

Fully immerse yourself in that moment, appreciating it to the fullest.

Savoring the small joys of life trains your mind to notice and cherish the fleeting moments of happiness that often go unnoticed. It encourages mindfulness and deepens your appreciation for life's simple pleasures.

Integration into Your Life

Gratitude is a practice that becomes more meaningful with consistency. To incorporate it into your daily life, consider the following tips:

Set a daily reminder: Use a phone app or a physical alarm to prompt your gratitude practice at a consistent time each day.

Share gratitude: Encourage family members or friends to join you in a gratitude practice, creating a supportive community of positivity.

Expand your focus: As you progress, challenge yourself to find gratitude in challenging or difficult situations, cultivating resilience and perspective.

As you embrace gratitude, you'll discover that it is not just a fleeting emotion but a way of life a lens through which you see the world. It offers a sanctuary of joy and contentment amidst the cacophony of daily life, reminding you of the profound abundance that surrounds you. Gratitude is a beacon that guides you to a more fulfilled and harmonious existence, one grateful moment at a time.

Inspiration from Real-Life Transformations

In the realm of mental health, where each individual's journey is as unique as their fingerprints, stories of transformation hold an unparalleled power. Throughout this chapter, you'll have the privilege of stepping into the shoes of real people who have embarked on their own quests for mental well-being. Their stories are not only testaments to the profound change that can be achieved but also a source of inspiration a reminder that the path to a happier, healthier you is not a distant dream but a tangible reality.

The Realization of Change

Life, in its relentless whirlwind, often presents us with challenges that seem insurmountable. The weight of anxiety, the darkness of depression, and the pressure of daily life can converge to create a sense of hopelessness. In those moments, it's easy to believe that change is beyond our grasp. Yet, these stories illuminate the truth that change is not only possible but achievable.

Consider Sarah's journey. She once grappled with crippling anxiety, her mind a tempest of worry and fear. The simplest tasks felt like insurmountable mountains. But, with a determined spirit, she ventured into the world of mindfulness. Through mindful breathing and self-compassion practices, she discovered a newfound sense of calm and control. Anxiety, while still a visitor in her life, no longer held the reins. Sarah's transformation demonstrates that even the most entrenched challenges can be met with resilience and the right tools.

The Journey, not a Destination

It's essential to understand that the mental health exercises presented in this book are not quick fixes or magical incantations. They are tools, much like a sculptor's chisel or a painter's brush, that require patience, practice, and persistence. Just as physical exercise gradually strengthens the body, these exercises fortify the mind over time.

Imagine John's story, a man who battled with the relentless grip of depression. He embraced journaling for self-discovery, using carefully curated prompts to explore his inner world. The act of writing became his sanctuary, a place to lay bare his thoughts and emotions without judgment. Over weeks and months, he observed patterns in his thinking and discovered the roots of his depression. Journaling became his compass, guiding him toward healthier thought patterns and a deeper understanding of himself. John's story reminds us that transformation is a journey, not a destination. Each journal entry was a step closer to his happier self.

Every Small Step Matters

In the pursuit of better mental health, it's crucial to understand that progress is rarely linear. It's not about making giant leaps or grand gestures but about taking small, deliberate steps each day. These steps, no matter how seemingly insignificant, accumulate like droplets of water forming a river. Each moment dedicated to your mental well-being contributes to the tapestry of your transformation.

Take Maria, for example. She grappled with the overwhelming stress of her demanding job and family responsibilities. Mindful breathing became her lifeline. It was a practice she could turn to during the chaos of her day. Inhale, exhale moments of mindfulness amidst the storm. Over time, her stress lessened, and she felt more centered and resilient. Maria's journey reminds us that even on the most challenging days, when motivation wanes, the simple act of trying is a triumph.

Your Unique Journey

As you navigate the chapters that follow, each dedicated to a specific mental health exercise, remember that your journey is unique. What resonates with one person may not align with another, and that's perfectly valid. The diversity of experiences and preferences is not only accepted but celebrated. Your journey is a canvas, waiting for your brush strokes of mindfulness, journaling, relaxation, and gratitude to create a masterpiece that is distinctly yours.

Support Along the Way

In closing, know that you are not alone on this transformative journey. We are here to guide and support you at every twist and turn. The wisdom and experiences shared within these pages are your companions. They offer insights, encouragement, and a sense of community on your path to better mental health.

So, as you embark on this journey, take a moment to embrace the stories of real-life transformations. These stories are a testament to the potential within each of us the potential to reshape the narrative of our mental well-being. Together, we'll delve deeper into each practical mental health exercise, providing you with the tools and knowledge to integrate them effectively into your life.

Your path to a happier, healthier you begin here, and we're honored to be a part of your journey. Let's take this transformative journey one exercise at a time, with the understanding that change is not just a distant dream but a tangible reality within your reach.

Understanding the Power of Positive Affirmations

Positive affirmations are not just empty words; they have a scientific basis for their effectiveness in building resilience and self-belief. When used correctly, they can rewire your thought patterns and boost your confidence. Here's how it works:

1. The Brain's Plasticity: Your brain is constantly evolving and adapting. It has the ability to form new neural connections and reorganize itself. Positive affirmations can help create new, positive neural pathways, weakening the old, negative ones.

2. Overcoming Negativity Bias: The human brain has a natural tendency to focus on negative thoughts and experiences. This is known as the negativity bias. Positive affirmations act as a counterbalance, shifting your focus towards more positive thoughts and beliefs.

3. Confidence and Self-Belief: Affirmations are like seeds planted in your subconscious. With repetition, they can sprout into strong, self-affirming beliefs. This increased self-belief can help you face challenges and setbacks with resilience.

4. Stress Reduction: Using affirmations can reduce the production of stress-related hormones like cortisol. This, in turn, can enhance your ability to cope with stress and adversity.

Crafting Affirmations that Resonate

The effectiveness of affirmations lies in their personalization. Here's a step-by-step guide to creating your own affirmations:

1. Identify Your Goals: Determine what areas of your life you want to improve or where you need more resilience. This could be self-esteem, stress management, or any other aspect.

2. Make Them Positive: Phrase your affirmations in a positive and present-tense manner. Instead of saying, "I am not afraid of failure," say, "I am confident in my abilities."

3. Keep Them Short and Specific: Make your affirmations concise and specific. This makes them easier to remember and focus on.

4. Use Emotion-Driven Language: Inject emotion into your affirmations. The more emotionally charged they are, the more impact they have on your subconscious mind.

5. Believe in Them: You must believe that your affirmations are true or can become true. This belief fuels their effectiveness.

Making Affirmations Part of Your Daily Life

Creating affirmations is just the beginning; integrating them into your daily routine is key to their effectiveness. Here's how:

1. Morning Routine: Start your day with a few minutes of repeating your affirmations. This sets a positive tone for the day ahead.

2. Sticky Notes: Write your affirmations on sticky notes and place them where you'll see them often—on your bathroom mirror, computer screen, or fridge.

3. Visualization: Along with reciting your affirmations, visualize yourself living the reality described in them. This can make them even more powerful.

4. Affirmation Journal: Maintain a journal to track your progress. Write down how you felt before and after using your affirmations.

5. Consistency: Consistency is key. Make affirmations a daily practice, even when you don't feel like it. Over time, they will become second nature.

Testimonial: Maria's Journey to Self-Love

Maria's story is a testament to the transformative power of positive affirmations. Despite the trauma she endured, she found a path to healing and self-love through the consistent practice of affirmations. Her story serves as inspiration, showing that with dedication and belief in oneself, anyone can build resilience and overcome even the most challenging obstacles.

Maria's story is a powerful testament to the transformative force of positive affirmations in the context of healing and personal growth. As a survivor of trauma, she grappled with the enduring impact of her past experiences, including self-doubt and negative self-talk. Through the practice of positive affirmations, Maria embarked on a remarkable journey of healing, self-rediscovery, and resilience.

The Shadows of Trauma

Maria's trauma left indelible scars, both physical and emotional. It cast long shadows over her self-esteem and self-worth. For years, she carried the heavy burden of self-doubt and a pervasive inner voice that whispered unworthiness.

The Search for Healing

Seeking respite from her internal struggles, Maria explored various avenues for healing. She attended therapy, engaged in support groups, and read self-help books. While these efforts provided some relief, she was still plagued by the relentless negative narrative within her mind.

The Discovery of Positive Affirmations

One day, while browsing a bookstore, Maria stumbled upon a book on positive affirmations. The concept intrigued her - the idea that simple, positive statements could rewire her thought patterns and help her cultivate self-worth. She decided to give it a try.

The Daily Practice Begins

Maria began her daily practice of positive affirmations. Each morning, she stood in front of her mirror, looked into her own eyes, and recited affirmations such as "I am worthy of love and happiness," "I am strong and resilient," and "I believe in myself." At first, it felt awkward and contrived, but she persevered.

Challenging the Inner Critic

The real power of positive affirmations emerged when Maria started challenging her inner critic. Every time a negative thought crept in, she countered it with a positive affirmation. Over time, the affirmations became a shield against the onslaught of self-doubt and criticism.

Cultivating Self-Compassion

Positive affirmations also played a crucial role in cultivating self-compassion. Maria learned to treat herself with the same kindness and understanding she would offer to a dear friend. She realized that her worthiness was not contingent on past experiences but an inherent part of her being.

Reclaiming Self-Worth

As Maria continued her practice, she began to notice subtle but significant shifts in her self-perception. She started to believe the affirmations she repeated daily. Her sense of self-worth grew stronger, and she felt a newfound confidence in her ability to face life's challenges.

Resilience in the Face of Triggers

Maria's journey wasn't without its triggers. Certain situations would still bring back memories of her trauma, and occasionally, the negative self-talk would resurface. But she had developed resilience through her affirmations, a powerful tool to help her bounce back from setbacks.

Sharing Her Transformation

Maria's transformation was nothing short of remarkable, and she felt compelled to share her experience with others who might be battling their own inner demons. She started leading workshops on positive affirmations and self-empowerment, helping others harness the same transformative force that had changed her life.

The Ongoing Journey

Maria's journey continues as a testament to the enduring nature of self-discovery and healing. She understands that affirmations are not a one-time fix but an ongoing practice. They are her allies in the ongoing process of growth and resilience.

Maria's story is a beacon of hope for those who have suffered trauma and wrestled with self-doubt. Her journey illustrates that, no matter the depth of one's wounds, the practice of positive affirmations can be a transformative force. Through affirmations, Maria reclaimed her sense of self-worth and resilience, demonstrating that healing and personal growth are possible for anyone willing to take that first step towards self-affirmation and self-love.

The Mind-Body Connection

The relationship between physical activity and mental health is not coincidental; it's rooted in science. Here's how exercise can positively impact your emotional well-being:

1. Brain Chemicals: When you exercise, your brain releases chemicals like endorphins and serotonin, often referred to as "feel-good" hormones. These chemicals can improve your mood and reduce symptoms of depression and anxiety.

2. Stress Reduction: Physical activity reduces the production of stress hormones like cortisol. It helps your body and mind relax, making you more resilient to stressors.

3. Cognitive Benefits: Exercise increases blood flow to the brain, enhancing cognitive function and memory. This can help with clarity of thought and decision-making.

4. Social Interaction: Many forms of exercise, such as group fitness classes or team sports, provide opportunities for social interaction, which can combat feelings of loneliness and improve overall mental well-being.

5. Routine and Structure: Establishing a regular exercise routine can provide structure and purpose in your daily life, which is especially valuable when dealing with mental health challenges.

Finding Joy in Movement

Exercise doesn't have to mean grueling workouts at the gym. It can take many forms, and the key is to find activities that you genuinely enjoy. Here's how to make physical activity a part of your life:

1. Choose Activities You Love: Whether it's dancing, hiking, swimming, or playing a sport, find activities that bring you joy. When you enjoy what you're doing, you're more likely to stick with it.

2. Start Small: If you're new to exercise, begin with short, manageable sessions. Gradually increase the intensity and duration as you build your fitness level.

3. Set Realistic Goals: Define clear, achievable fitness goals. This gives you a sense of purpose and accomplishment as you progress.

4. Make It Social: Exercise with friends or join group classes. Social support can be a powerful motivator.

5. Mix It Up: Variety keeps things interesting. Rotate between different activities to prevent boredom.

Sustainable Routines for Mental Well-being

Consistency is key when it comes to reaping the mental health benefits of exercise. Here are some strategies to help you make physical activity a habit:

1. Schedule It: Treat exercise like any other important appointment. Block out time in your calendar for it.

2. Find Accountability: Share your exercise goals with a friend or family member who can hold you accountable.

3. Track Your Progress: Maintain a workout journal to record your achievements. Seeing your progress can be motivating.

4. Reward Yourself: Celebrate your fitness milestones with small rewards. This reinforces the positive association with exercise.

5. Be Patient: Remember that the mental health benefits of exercise may take time to fully manifest. Be patient with yourself and your progress.

Testimonial: David's Triumph Over Depression

David's story serves as a powerful reminder of the potential of physical activity to aid in the management and overcoming of mental health challenges. Through regular exercise, he not only found relief from depression but also discovered a renewed sense of purpose and well-being. His journey showcases the profound impact that exercise can have on mental health and offers hope to others facing similar struggles.

Chapter 13 - Crafting Your Personalized Mental Health Plan

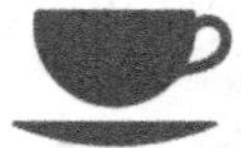

In the final section, readers are encouraged to take charge of their emotional well-being by crafting a personalized mental health plan. By reflecting on their unique goals, needs, and preferences, readers can tailor a plan that aligns with their individual circumstances. We provide a practical template and offer guidance on setting achievable objectives and integrating mental health exercises into daily life.

Why Personalization Matters

No two individuals are alike, and this holds true for our mental health needs as well. What works wonders for one person might not be as effective for another. Recognizing this uniqueness is the first step towards building a plan that truly aligns with your individual circumstances.

Reflecting on Your Goals, Needs, and Preferences

Start by asking yourself some fundamental questions:

What are your primary mental health goals? Is it to reduce stress, manage anxiety, overcome depression, or simply enhance overall well-being?

What are your specific needs? Consider your current emotional state. Do you require more self-care, social connection, or professional support?

What are your preferences? Think about the methods and activities that resonate with you. Are you drawn to mindfulness meditation, physical exercise, creative pursuits, or a combination of these?

Creating Your Mental Health Plan

Here's a practical template to help you create your personalized mental health plan:

Identify Your Objectives: Clearly define your mental health goals. Be specific and measurable. For instance, instead of saying "I want to reduce stress," try "I will practice deep breathing exercises for 10 minutes every day to reduce my stress levels by 20% in the next month."

Choose Your Activities: Based on your needs and preferences, select activities or strategies that align with your goals. These could include meditation, yoga, journaling, spending time with loved ones, or seeking professional therapy.

Set a Schedule: Determine when and how often you'll engage in these activities. Consistency is key. Incorporate them into your daily or weekly routine.

Track Your Progress: Keep a journal to record your experiences and track your progress. Note how each activity makes you feel and whether it's helping you achieve your goals.

Adjust as Needed: Life is dynamic, and so are our mental health needs. Periodically review your plan, reassess your objectives, and make adjustments as necessary. Don't be afraid to seek new strategies if something isn't working for you.

Integrating Mental Health into Daily Life

The key to a successful mental health plan is integration into your daily life. Make it a habit, just like brushing your teeth or having breakfast. Small, consistent efforts can lead to significant improvements over time.

Remember, there's no one-size-fits-all solution to mental health. Your journey is unique, and your plan should reflect that. Be patient with yourself, and don't hesitate to seek professional guidance if needed. With dedication and a well-crafted plan, you're taking a significant step toward a healthier, happier you.

Making Exercise a Habit: Sustainable Routines for Mental Well-being

Consistency is key when it comes to reaping the mental health benefits of exercise. In this chapter, we will explore strategies to help you make physical activity a regular and sustainable part of your life, paving the way for improved mental well-being.

1. SCHEDULE IT: PRIORITIZE Your Health

Treat exercise like any other essential appointment. Just as you wouldn't cancel an important meeting or doctor's visit, block out time in your calendar for exercise. This simple act of scheduling can help you prioritize your health.

2. Find Accountability: Share Your Goals

Accountability can be a powerful motivator. Share your exercise goals with a friend or family member who can hold you accountable. Knowing that someone is cheering you on and expecting you to follow through can be a strong incentive to stick with your exercise routine.

3. Track Your Progress: Celebrate Achievements

Maintain a workout journal to record your achievements. Whether it's running an extra mile, lifting heavier weights, or simply completing your daily workout, seeing your progress in black and white can be highly motivating. It provides tangible evidence of your commitment and growth.

4. Reward Yourself: Reinforce Positivity

Celebrate your fitness milestones with small rewards. Treat yourself to something you enjoy after a successful workout or achieving a specific goal. This positive reinforcement creates a pleasurable association with exercise, making you more likely to continue.

5. Be Patient: Mental Health Benefits Take Time

Exercise is a powerful tool for enhancing mental well-being, but the benefits may not be immediate. Be patient with yourself and your progress. Understand that the mental health benefits of exercise, such as reduced stress and improved mood, may take time to fully manifest. Stick with your routine, and over time, you'll likely notice positive changes in your mental state.

Testimonial: David's Triumph Over Depression

David's story serves as a powerful testament to the potential of physical activity in managing and overcoming mental health challenges. Struggling with depression, David embarked on a journey of regular exercise. Through dedication and commitment, he not only found relief from his depression but also discovered a renewed sense of purpose and overall well-being.

David's story showcases the profound impact that exercise can have on mental health. It offers hope and inspiration to others facing similar struggles, demonstrating that with perseverance and a well-structured exercise routine, one can triumph over mental health challenges and find a path to a brighter future.

DAVID'S JOURNEY IS a compelling testament to the potent alliance between physical activity and mental health. As a software engineer battling depression, he embarked on a transformative path of healing, resilience, and self-discovery through regular exercise.

The Shadows of Depression

Depression had cast a long shadow over David's life. The demands of his job, coupled with the isolation of working remotely, exacerbated his feelings of sadness and hopelessness. He struggled to find joy in the activities he once loved and often felt trapped in a cycle of negative thoughts.

The Turning Point

One day, David reached a turning point. He realized that he needed to take action to improve his mental health. Seeking an escape from the relentless grip of depression, he turned to exercise as a potential solution.

The Power of Physical Activity

David started with small steps, going for short walks in his neighborhood. The fresh air and movement provided a welcome break from the confines of his home office. Gradually, he incorporated more structured physical activities into his routine, including jogging and cycling.

The Brain-Boosting Effects

As he became more physically active, David began to experience the profound effects on his mental health. Exercise triggered the release of endorphins, the body's natural mood lifters, helping to alleviate the cloud of sadness that had shrouded him for so long. He found that after each workout, his mind felt clearer, and his mood improved.

A Sense of Achievement

Exercise provided David with a sense of achievement that had been lacking in his life. Setting and achieving fitness goals, no matter how small, gave him a sense of purpose and direction. It was a tangible reminder that he had the power to make positive changes in his life.

Connecting with Others

David also discovered the social benefits of exercise. He joined a local running club and started participating in group fitness classes. These interactions not only boosted his mood but also fostered a sense of belonging and camaraderie, combating the isolation he had felt.

Stress Reduction and Sleep Improvement

Exercise served as a powerful stress reducer for David. It helped him manage the daily pressures of his job more effectively, and he found that he slept better at night, which in turn had a positive impact on his overall mental well-being.

Resilience in the Face of Challenges

David's journey wasn't without its challenges. There were days when depression tried to pull him back into its grip. However, he had developed resilience through his exercise routine. On his most challenging days, he leaned on the discipline and determination he had cultivated.

A Lifelong Commitment

David's journey continues as a lifelong commitment to his mental health. He understands that exercise is not a panacea but a vital component of his well-being. It's a journey of self-care, self-compassion, and self-discovery.

Sharing His Triumph

David's transformation inspired him to share his journey with others. He started volunteering at local mental health organizations, offering support and guidance to individuals battling depression. His story became a source of inspiration for those seeking solace and healing through physical activity.

David's story is a testament to the remarkable potential of exercise in managing and overcoming mental health challenges. It illustrates that, no matter the depths of despair, the simple act of moving one's body can be a catalyst for healing and transformation. Through regular exercise, David not only managed his depression but discovered a profound sense of resilience and self-empowerment, showcasing the profound connection between physical and mental well-being.

Chapter 14 - The Empowered Pursuit of Emotional Well-being

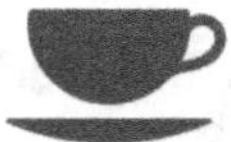

In the concluding chapter of our journey, we arrive at the heart of the matter: the empowered pursuit of emotional well-being. Throughout this book, we have explored the significance of mental health exercises, their transformative potential, and the profound impact they can have on our lives. Now, as we conclude, it is essential to recognize that the pursuit of emotional well-being is not merely a passive endeavor but an empowered and active journey.

Recognizing Your Inner Strength

Embracing emotional well-being begins with recognizing the inner strength that resides within each of us. It is the understanding that we possess the power to shape our emotional landscape, to navigate the complexities of life with resilience, and to cultivate a positive and balanced mindset. This recognition is the first step towards an empowered pursuit of emotional well-being.

The Lifelong Journey

It's important to acknowledge that emotional well-being is not a fixed destination but a lifelong journey. This journey is dynamic and ever-evolving, characterized by growth, self-discovery, and continuous improvement. It invites us to explore the depths of our emotions, to confront challenges with courage, and to adapt to the ebb and flow of life with grace.

Taking Ownership of Your Well-being

Empowerment in the pursuit of emotional well-being comes from taking ownership of your well-being. It means recognizing that you are the steward of your own mental health and that your choices, actions, and mindset profoundly influence your emotional state. It's about making intentional decisions that prioritize your emotional health and foster a positive outlook.

The Transformative Potential of Mental Health Exercises

Throughout this book, we've explored a wide range of mental health exercises mindfulness practices, journaling prompts, relaxation techniques, and more. These exercises serve as powerful tools on your journey towards emotional well-being. They are not mere activities but gateways to self-awareness, emotional regulation, and personal growth. By integrating these exercises into your daily life, you unlock their transformative potential.

Embracing Resilience and Balance

An empowered pursuit of emotional well-being involves embracing resilience and balance. Resilience allows you to bounce back from adversity, to weather life's storms with fortitude, and to emerge stronger from challenges. Balance ensures that you prioritize self-care, maintain healthy boundaries, and cultivate a harmonious life that supports your emotional well-being.

The Power of Connection and Support

While personal empowerment is vital, it's essential to recognize the power of connection and support. Emotional well-being is not a solitary endeavor but one that thrives in the context of meaningful relationships. Seek support from friends, family, or professionals when needed. Share your journey with others, for collective support can be a wellspring of strength.

Conclusion: Your Empowered Journey

As we conclude our exploration of the empowered pursuit of emotional well-being, remember that you are the author of your emotional narrative. You have the capacity to shape your emotional landscape, to overcome challenges, and to lead a life characterized by balance, resilience, and positivity. The pursuit of emotional well-being is a journey that unfolds one step at a time, one exercise at a time, and one mindful moment at a time.

May this concluding chapter serve as an invitation to embark on your empowered journey towards emotional well-being. Embrace the knowledge, tools, and exercises you've encountered in this book as companions on your path. Trust in your inner strength, and know that the pursuit of emotional well-being is a profoundly rewarding endeavor one that empowers you to live a life filled with emotional vitality, contentment, and fulfillment.

Testimonial: Sarah's Journey to Emotional Well-Being

My journey to emotional well-being has been a transformative one, and I wanted to share my story in the hopes that it might inspire others who are on a similar path.

For many years, I struggled with my emotions. Anxiety seemed to be my constant companion, and I often found myself overwhelmed by stress and self-doubt. The pressures of daily life, from work demands to personal responsibilities, had taken a toll on my mental and emotional health.

The Breaking Point

There came a point where I felt like I was on the verge of breaking. The weight of my emotions was suffocating, and I knew that I needed to make a change. It was during this time of crisis that I began to explore different avenues for improving my emotional well-being.

The Role of Mindfulness

One of the most transformative practices on my journey was mindfulness. It started with a simple meditation app I downloaded on a whim. I remember my first session; my mind was racing, and I felt a bit silly sitting in silence. But as I continued to practice, something incredible happened.

Finding Peace in the Present Moment

Mindfulness taught me the power of the present moment. It helped me see that so much of my anxiety was rooted in worrying about the future or ruminating on the past. By learning to be fully present in each moment, I discovered a profound sense of peace.

Embracing My Emotions

Another important aspect of my journey was learning to embrace my emotions, even the difficult ones. Instead of trying to suppress or avoid them, I learned to sit with my feelings, acknowledging them without judgment. This self-compassion was a revelation.

The Power of Connection

I also realized the importance of connection. Opening up to friends and family about my struggles allowed me to build a support system that I hadn't fully appreciated before. Their empathy and understanding became a source of strength.

Seeking Professional Help

In addition to self-help practices, I sought the guidance of a therapist. Talking to a professional helped me gain insights into the root causes of my anxiety and provided me with strategies to manage it effectively.

Small Steps, Big Changes

My journey to emotional well-being was not without its challenges. There were setbacks, moments when anxiety reared its head, and times when I doubted my progress. But I learned that healing is a process, and every small step forward was a victory.

A Brighter Tomorrow

Today, I can say that my emotional well-being has undergone a profound transformation. While I still have moments of anxiety, they no longer define me. I've learned to navigate my emotions with grace and resilience. I wake up each day with a sense of hope and gratitude, knowing that I have the tools to face whatever challenges come my way.

A Message of Hope

I share my story with the hope that it might inspire someone else who is struggling with their emotional well-being. You don't have to remain trapped in the cycle of anxiety and stress. There is a path to emotional well-being, and it begins with the decision to take that first step towards healing. You are stronger than you know, and there is a brighter tomorrow waiting for you.

This testimonial highlights the journey of an individual who struggled with emotional well-being and found hope and transformation through mindfulness, self-compassion, connection, and professional support. It emphasizes that healing is a process and offers a message of hope to others facing similar challenges.

Did you love *Mental Health and Well Being*? Then you should read *Secrets of Mount Kailash, Bermuda Triangle and the Lost City of Atlantis* by Jagdish Arora!

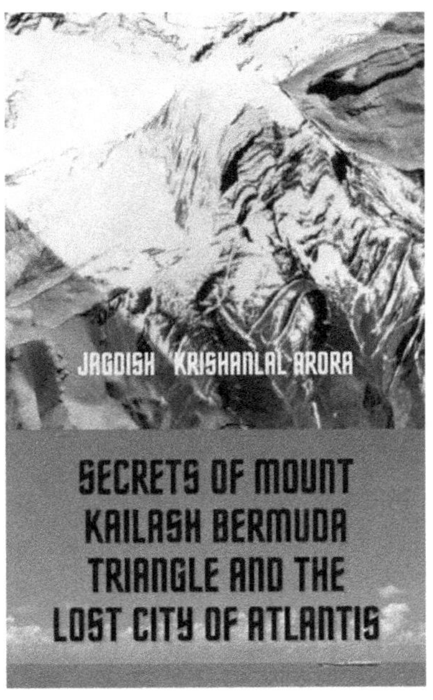

The book goes into the details on the mysteries surrounding Mount Kailash, Bermuda Triangle, and the Lost City of Atlantis. It is also a good book to read for people who like to travel to unknown and mysterious places in the mountains and jungles.

'Secrets of Mount Kailash, Bermuda Triangle, and the Lost City of Atlantis' invites you to explore the world's most intriguing mysteries. Embark on an exhilarating journey as explore the mystique of Mount Kailash's spiritual significance, the enigmatic Bermuda Triangle's tales of disappearances, and the legendary lost city of Atlantis. This book unearths ancient legends, modern investigations, and theories that shroud these place..Join us in uncovering the hidden truths, speculation, and wonder that surround these captivating phenomena."

Also by Jagdish Krishanlal Arora